Neurology
for the
House Officer

THIRD EDITION

Neurology
for the
House Officer

THIRD EDITION

Howard L. Weiner, M.D.
Associate in Medicine (Neurology)
Brigham and Women's Hospital
Associate Professor of Neurology
Harvard Medical School
Boston, Massachusetts

Lawrence P. Levitt, M.D.
Chief, Division of Neurology
Allentown Hospital and the Lehigh Valley Hospital Center
Allentown, Pennsylvania
Associate in Neurology
University of Pennsylvania School of Medicine
Clinical Assistant Professor of Neurology
Temple University School of Medicine
Philadelphia, Pennsylvania

WILLIAMS & WILKINS
Baltimore • London • Los Angeles • Sydney

Copyright ©, 1983
Williams & Wilkins
428 East Preston Street
Baltimore, MD 21202, U.S.A.

Made in the United States of America
Second Edition 1978

Library of Congress Cataloging in Publication Data

Weiner, Howard L.
  Neurology for the house officer.

  1. Nervous system—Diseases—Handbooks, manuals, etc. 2. Neurology—Hand-books, manuals, etc. I. Levitt, Lawrence P. II. Title. [DNLM: 1. Nervous system diseases. 2. Neurologic manifestations. WL 100 W424n]
RC355.W44 1983 616.8 83-16849
ISBN 0-683-08910-3

Composed and printed at the
Waverly Press, Inc.
Mt. Royal and Guilford Aves.
Baltimore, MD 21202, U.S.A.   88 89   10 9 8

Dedication

To our wives Mira and Eva

Foreword

Having spent my professional life in a teaching
hospital with a steady stream of students, house officers,
and residents, I have gradually become accustomed to the
varying neurological backgrounds of these young
physicians.

The neurologist and the internist exhibit significant
differences in approach. The internist is usually trained
to think physiologically in terms of the meaning and cause
of specific symptoms. The neurologist, on the other hand,
brings to the patient encounter not only his history and
general physical examination, but a special "neurological
examination". This special examination is designed more
to answer the question "Where is the lesion?" than "What
is wrong with the patient?".

In this country, most students and medical residents,
general practitioners, and internists do not develop
strong backgrounds in neurology. They therefore profit
less from their neurologic endeavors than they might.
Nevertheless, they are still required to care for patients
with nervous system disorders and are often significantly
insecure about treatment.

In attempting to deal with this problem, Howard L.
Weiner and Lawrence P. Levitt began compiling notes for
their lectures to small groups of students. This soon
became source material for future reference. The demand
for this material grew geometrically and was widely used
by students and residents. The need for a practical
manual was appreciated, and the authors began a more
systematic approach to problems with which they were

recurrently faced on the wards of a large teaching hospital. As fast as they could put the sections out, students, medical interns, and residents kept requesting them, and soon large numbers were being duplicated. The material was recognized for its practical and common sense approach to problems frequently encountered.

After an intensive effort to gather constructive suggestions, find unmet needs, and weed out unimportant material, the authors wrote the first edition of this handbook almost ten years ago.

Since its publication, Neurology for the House Officer has been enthusiastically received by physicians throughout the United States and has been published in several foreign language editions. It has become a standard guide for approaching neurologic problems and its format has been the impetus for the creation of an entire series of house officer manuals in a variety of specialties.

I am certain that the third edition of this handbook will continue to meet the practical needs of physicians who care for patients with nervous system disorders.

H. Richard Tyler, M.D.

About the Authors

Howard L. Weiner, M.D., is Associate in Medicine
(Neurology) at the Brigham and Women's Hospital and
Associate Professor of Neurology at Harvard Medical
School. He attended Dartmouth College and the University
of Colorado Medical School; he then interned at Chaim
Sheba Hospital, Tel Hashomer, Israel, and served as a
medical resident at the Beth Israel Hospital, Boston. Dr.
Weiner is currently involved in immunology and virology
research as applied to the nervous system, with a special
interest in multiple sclerosis.

Lawrence P. Levitt, M.D., is chief of the Division of
Neurology at Allentown Hospital and the Lehigh Valley
Hospital Center in Allentown, Pennsylvania, and is an
Associate in Neurology at the University of Pennsylvania
School of Medicine, and Clinical Assistant Professor of
Neurology at Temple University School of Medicine. A
graduate of Queens College, he then attended Cornell
Medical College as a Jonas Salk Scholar. Dr. Levitt
interned and was a first-year medical resident at Bellevue
Hospital and then spent two years in the Public Health
Service at the Encephalitis Research Center in Tampa,
Florida.

With a Foreword by H. Richard Tyler, M.D.

H. Richard Tyler, M.D. is Professor of Neurology at
Harvard Medical School, physician and Head of the Section
of Neurology at the Brigham and Women's Hospital. He
serves as Consultant in Neurology for the Beth Israel
Hospital, Children's Hospital Medical Center, and the West

Roxbury VA Hospital. His responsibilities have included
teaching of students, interns, and residents in the
Harvard Medical School for over 20 years. He serves as
Tutor in Neurology for the Harvard Medical School. Dr.
Tyler is the author of numerous articles relating to the
neurologic aspects of medical disease.

Preface

This manual is designed to help physicians properly recognize and treat neurologic disease. It is not meant to be a complete survey but an attempt to outline succinctly the important clinical information about common neurologic problems. In the third edition we have added new chapters on neurologic diagnosis (e.g., CAT scan, evoked potentials) and sleep disorders, updated references and treatment modalities, and included pertinent advances in neurologic diagnosis.

The approach is problem oriented: How to deal with a patient who is comatose, has a right hemiplegia, or is demented. We are most gratified by the widespread use the previous editions of the manual have received and hope the third edition continues to fill the need for a readable "carry in the pocket", practical reference to neurologic problems.

Howard L. Weiner, M.D.
Lawrence P. Levitt, M.D.

Acknowledgments

This manual was reviewed by students and house officers at the Harvard teaching hospitals of the Longwood Area Neurology Program. We are grateful to them for their encouragement, enthusiasm, and advice, and for identifying those neurologic problems and concepts most important to them. We would like to thank the following members of the neurology staff and house staff for their help and for reviewing parts of the manuscript: Doctors P. Barbour, C. Barlow, M. Biber, R. Brown, Jr., L. Caplan, D. Dawson, M. Dichter, N. Geschwind, D. Hafler, S. Hauser, S. Schachter, S. Tepper, H.R. Tyler, and K. Winston.

Contents

nature and degree of central
nervous system dysfunction.
This chapter presents an
approach to examining and evalu-
ating the comatose patient.

Chapter 1

Localization

One of the major features of neurological diagnosis is <u>localization of the lesion</u> in the nervous system. This approach is needed if one is to consistently arrive at reasonable diagnoses. Anatomic orientation is not merely an intellectual exercise; knowing where the lesion is will often tell what it is, help guide in management, and be crucial in deciding on diagnostic procedures. For example:

PURE MOTOR HEMIPLEGIA (Chapter 6)

The nature of its anatomy defines the vascular lesion as a lacune and means arteriography, anticoagulation or surgery are usually not indicated.

MULTIPLE SCLEROSIS

One needs multiple lesions in the nervous system and a history of exacerbations and remissions for the diagnosis. When patients are misdiagnosed as having multiple sclerosis, there was often only one anatomical lesion.

HYSTERICAL SYMPTOMS

Hysteria is suspected when symptoms and/or signs do not fit anatomical rules.

FOOT-DROP

Foot drop can be seen with peripheral nerve,

spinal cord, or hemisphere disease; one must decide where the dysfunction is before beginning investigation.

Knowledge of detailed neuroanatomy is usually not needed to decide whether the lesion is cortical, subcortical, in the brainstem, spinal cord, peripheral nerve, or muscle. When necessary, anatomical localization can be refined -- first with the help of this manual, later with textbooks. If after completing the history and physical examination the physician begins his analysis by asking "Where is the lesion?", he will have overcome the major obstacle in making neurologic diagnoses.

REFERENCE

1.   Haymaker W: <u>Bing's Local Diagnosis in Neurological Disease</u>. St. Louis, C.V. Mosby Co., 1969.

Chapter 2

Right Hemiplegia

When examining a patient with right hemiplegia (paralysis) or right hemiparesis (weakness), establish whether the lesion is cortical, subcortical, in the brainstem, or spinal cord (Fig. 1).

IS THE LESION CORTICAL?

1. Test the patient carefully for <u>aphasia</u>. Have him name objects (e.g., pen, tie, watch), repeat ("no if's, and's, or but's"), read (a magazine or newspaper) and check for comprehension. Listen carefully to spontaneous speech for aphasic errors. Remember, in nearly all right-handed and most left-handed people, the left hemisphere is dominant for speech (see chapter 4, <u>Aphasia</u>).

2. Check for <u>cortical sensory loss</u>. Test position sense, point localization, graphesthesia (write numbers on the palm), and stereognosis (using a coin, comb, or pen).

3. Are the <u>face and arm more involved than the leg</u> (suggesting middle cerebral artery territory), or is the <u>leg more involved</u> (anterior cerebral)?

4. Is there <u>eye deviation</u>? Eyes deviate toward the hemisphere involved and away from the hemiparesis in cortical lesions (see Fig. 5, Chapter 28).

5.   Check carefully for a <u>field defect</u>. Have patient
identify fingers presented simultaneously in
peripheral fields. <u>Note</u>: Field defects and
"cortical-type" eye deviation may be found in
subcortical lesions and must be interpreted in the
context of other findings. The presence of seizures,
cortical sensory less, or aphasia will often resolve
this issue.

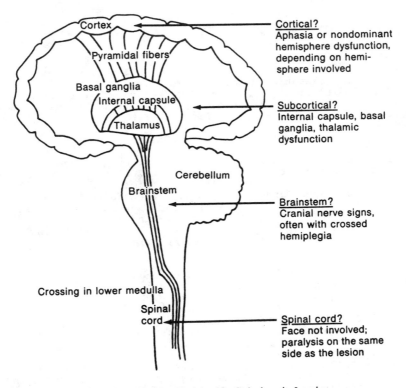

Is the lesion

Cortical?
Aphasia or nondominant
hemisphere dysfunction,
depending on hemi-
sphere involved

Subcortical?
Internal capsule, basal
ganglia, thalamic
dysfunction

Brainstem?
Cranial nerve signs,
often with crossed
hemiplegia

Spinal cord?
Face not involved;
paralysis on the same
side as the lesion

FIGURE 1 Right (left) hemiplegia

6.   Has the hemiparesis been associated with a seizure
     suggesting a cortical focus? Has the patient had
     seizures in the same distribution as the weakness?

              OR IS THE LESION SUBCORTICAL?

     Subcortical structures include the internal capsule,
basal ganglia (globus pallidus and putamen), and thalamus.

1.   Are <u>face, arm, and leg equally involved</u>
     (characteristic of lesions in the internal capsule)?

2.   Are there dystonic postures (seen with lesions of the
     basal ganglia)?

3.   Is there a <u>dense sensory loss</u> to pinprick and touch
     in face, arm, and leg (seen with thalamic lesions)
     associated with the hemiplegia? The latter is due to
     involvement of the adjacent internal capsule.

4.   Is there <u>eye deviation</u> or a field defect as seen in
     cortical lesions?

              IS THE LESION IN THE LEFT BRAINSTEM?

1.   Look for <u>crossed hemiplegia,</u> a classic feature of
     brainstem lesions. Right hemiplegia from a
     left-sided brainstem lesion often produces left-sided
     brainstem signs (e.g., left-sided dysmetria or
     cranial nerve palsies) at the level of the lesion.

2.   Check for <u>cerebellar signs</u>: finger-to-nose ataxia,
     difficulty with rapid alternating movements in the
     limbs, difficulty walking heel-to-toe (tandem gait).
     Remember -- limb ataxia is almost always on the same
     side as the lesion, so a left brainstem lesion gives
     left limb ataxia. Do <u>not</u> misinterpret weakness for
     ataxia.

3.   Note <u>nystagmus</u>. This is usually more marked when
     the patient gazes toward the side of the lesion.

4.   Check for <u>hearing loss</u> in the left ear.

5.   Check carefully for <u>sensory findings</u>: a
     characteristic finding is pain, temperature and
     corneal loss on the left side of the face

(involvement of descending tract of V) with pain and temperature loss on the right side of the body (spinothalamic tract). (See Fig. 9, Chapter 28)

6.   Note <u>dysarthria</u> and <u>difficulty with swallowing</u>. Pseudobulbar palsy, often secondary to multiple bilateral vascular lesions above the brainstem, also causes dysarthria and dysphagia. The patient with pseudobulbar palsy, though, usually has a hyperactive rather than a decreased gag, brisk jaw jerk, emotional lability, and a history of previous strokes.

7.   Check for abnormal <u>eye movements</u>. For example, patients with right hemiplegia secondary to left brainstem lesions may have trouble gazing to the left (See Fig. 5, Chapter 28) or in getting the left eye to cross the midline when looking to the right (internuclear ophthalmoplegia). (See Fig. 10, Chapter 28)

8.   Tongue deviation is to the left with lesions of the left twelfth nerve or its nucleus, since the stronger right-sided hypoglossus muscle pushes the tongue to the left. Left-sided lesions above the nucleus (including the cortex) may cause tongue deviation to the right, since supranuclear innervation is crossed.

OR IS THE LESION IN THE SPINAL CORD?

1.   The <u>face</u> is not involved. Language function and cranial nerves are not involved.

2.   <u>Paralysis</u> is on the same side as the lesion. <u>Pinprick and temperature</u> loss on the opposite side (Brown-Séquard syndrome) may be seen. (See Fig. 8, Chapter 28.)

3.   A <u>sensory level</u> to pinprick or vibration may be present.

4.   <u>Bladder</u> and bowel disturbances are common.

Chapter 3

Left Hemiplegia

When examining a patient with a left hemiplegia, nondominant hemisphere function rather than aphasia testing is stressed. The remainder of cortical, subcortical, brainstem, and spinal cord testing is the same.

ARE THERE NONDOMINANT HEMISPHERE FINDINGS?

1. Check for <u>inattention</u>. Does the patient ignore his left side, the left side of the room, or the left side of a picture? Check for <u>extinction</u> by double simultaneous sensory or visual stimulation (touch both his hands at once and ask which was touched; have patient identify fingers presented simultaneously in peripheral fields).

2. Check for <u>denial</u> or "<u>unconcern</u>". Does the patient deny that anything is wrong, or does he, despite awareness of his hemiplegia, show little concern? Sometimes, a patient will not recognize his own left hand when it is lifted in front of him.

3. Test for <u>constructional apraxia</u>. Have the patient attempt to copy a simple diagram (e.g., a cube) or designs made with tongue blades. Have him draw a clock and fill in the numbers.

4. <u>Does he have difficulty dressing</u> (dressing apraxia)?

5.   Check for spatial disorientation by leading the patient from his room: Can he find his way back? Have him analyze a picture. Check topography by asking him directions about local travel.

6.   Is there impersistence at a task? Can he hold his tongue out or maintain an "ahhh"?

7.   Is there an acute confusional state, as has been reported in some patients with non-dominant hemisphere strokes?

REFERENCES

1.   Critchley M: The Parietal Lobes. New York, Hafner Publishing Co., 1969.
2.   Denny-Brown D, Chambers RA: The parietal lobe and behavior. Res Publ Assoc Res Nerv Ment Dis 36:35, 1958.
3.   Fisher CM: Left hemiplegia and motor impersistence. J Nerv Ment Dis 123:201, 1956.
4.   Mesulam M-M, Waxman S, Geschwind N, et al.: Acute confusional states with right middle cerebral artery infarctions. J Neurol Neurosurg Psych 39:84, 1976.

Chapter 4

Aphasia

Aphasia is a disorder of language; the aphasic patient uses language incorrectly or comprehends it imperfectly. The dysarthric patient, on the other hand, articulates poorly, but his grammar and word choice are correct. Aphasia must be recognized clinically because it localizes the lesion to the cortex (or immediately under the cortex) and to the left hemisphere. There are three exceptions: (1) Some (less than 50%) left-handed people use the right hemisphere for speech; (2) Anomic aphasias may result from metabolic disorders or space-occupying lesions with pressure effects; (3) Thalamic lesions, especially on the left, may produce aphasia. Since different types of aphasia may imply different etiologies, the clinician must first be able to recognize that aphasia exists and then to characterize it.

ANATOMY OF APHASIA

Language "ability" is a function of the left hemisphere for almost all right-handed and for most left-handed individuals. The anatomic components of language are located primarily in the distribution of the middle cerebral artery surrounding the Sylvian and Rolandic fissures. Speech production involves four regions in this area, moving from posterior to anterior. Thus, speech connections exist between Wernicke's area (W) or the posterior part of the first temporal gyrus; the angular gyrus (AG); the arcuate fasciculus (AF); and Broca's area (B) or the posterior third frontal gyrus.

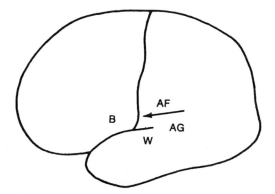

Wernicke's area lies next to the primary auditory cortex and involves the "understanding" of auditory input as language and monitors speech output. It is connected with the angular gyrus, a center for integrating sensory and other association information.

The arcuate fasciculus is a white matter tract leading to Broca's area, which in turn is responsible for the motor part or "production" of language. Broca's area translates the information carried from other speech areas into phonation and actual speech.

FIVE TYPES OF APHASIA

Broca's Aphasia

The lesion is in or near Broca's area.

1.   Speech is slow, nonfluent, produced with great effort, and poorly articulated. There is marked reduction in total speech, which may be "telegraphic" with the omission of small words or endings.

2.   Comprehension of written and verbal speech is good.

3.   Repetition of single words may be good, though it is done with great effort; phrase repetition is poor, especially phrases containing small function words (e.g., "no, if's, and's, or but's").

4.   The patient always writes in an aphasic manner.

5. <u>Object naming</u> is usually poor, although it may be better than spontaneous speech.

6. <u>Hemiparesis</u> (usually greater in the arm than the leg) is present, as the motor cortex is close to Broca's area.

7. The patient is <u>aware</u> of his deficit; he is frustrated and frequently depressed.

8. Interestingly, the patient may be able to hum a melody normally. Curses or other ejaculatory speech may be well articulated.

Wernicke's Aphasia

The lesion is in or near Wernicke's area.

1. <u>Speech</u> is <u>fluent</u> with normal rhythm and articulation, but it conveys information poorly because of circumlocutions, use of empty words and incorrect words (paraphasic errors).

2. The patient uses wrong words and sounds -- i.e., makes <u>paraphasic errors</u> ("treen" for train; "here is my clover" for here is my hand).

3. The patient is unable to <u>comprehend</u> written or verbal speech.

4. The content of <u>writing</u> is abnormal, as is speech, though the penmanship may be good.

5. <u>Repetition</u> is poor.

6. <u>Object naming</u> is poor.

7. <u>Hemiparesis</u> is mild or absent, since the lesion is far from the motor cortex. A hemianopsia or quadrantanopsia may be present.

8. Patients may not realize the nature of their deficit and usually are not depressed in the acute stage.

Conduction Aphasia

This is due to a temporal or parietal lesion involving the arcuate fasciculus and/or connecting fibers "disconnecting" Wernicke's and Broca's area.

1. Speech is fluent but conveys information imperfectly. Paraphasic errors are common.

2. The patient can comprehend spoken or written phrases containing small grammatical words.

3. Repetition is severely affected, especially for phrases containing small grammatical words.

4. There is difficulty naming objects.

5. Written language is impaired, though penmanship is preserved.

6. Hemiparesis, if present, is usually mild.

Anomic Aphasia

1. This type of aphasia may be seen with small lesions in the angular gyrus, toxic or metabolic encephalopathies, or with focal space-occupying lesions far from the speech area, but which exert pressure effects. It is the least localizing of the aphasias and should prompt a serious search for reversible, metabolic causes.

2. Speech is fluent but conveys information poorly because of paraphasic errors and circumlocutions (written language is impaired in the same way). Even though this aphasia is termed anomic aphasia (difficulty in naming objects), anomia is not unique to this type of aphasia.

3. The patient can understand both written and spoken speech.

4. There is no hemiplegia.

5. Comprehension and repetition are normal, although these may be difficult to assess in a patient who is confused.

Global Aphasia

This type of aphasia is seen with large lesions affecting both Wernicke's and Broca's areas. Hemiparesis occurs, plus inability to comprehend and to speak. Global aphasia is seen with large infarcts in the middle cerebral artery territory and is often due to occlusion of the left internal carotid artery or trunk of the middle cerebral artery.

Other Aphasic Syndromes

Broca's, Wernicke's, conduction, and global aphasias involve repetition difficulty because the lesion(s) involve the speech area in the perisylvian region. Less commonly, aphasias occur due to lesions located outside the perisylvian region, in "borderzone" areas. Aphasic syndromes, such as isolation of the speech area, transcortical motor aphasia, and transcortical sensory aphasia have been described (see references for details). Transcortical aphasias may occur after prolonged hypotension or hypoxia, e.g., after cardiac arrest. These patients often repeat and read well but have diminished fluency (anterior borderzone lesions) or comprehend poorly (posterior borderzone lesions).

EXAMINATION OF THE APHASIC PATIENT

It must first be established whether the patient is in fact aphasic; then determine the nature of the aphasia. Remember, it may be difficult to determine if an inattentive or confused patient is aphasic.

1. Listen to speech output. Is it fluent or nonfluent? If fluent, the lesion is posterior; if nonfluent, it usually is anterior.

2. Can the patient read and write with no errors? If so, he is not aphasic.

3. Is there hemiparesis? If so, the lesion is anterior, involving the motor area.

4. To delineate the various types of fluent aphasias, check to see if the patient can repeat, comprehend, and name.

- Wernicke's: cannot repeat or comprehend: names poorly

- Conduction: cannot repeat but can comprehend; names poorly

- Anomic: can both repeat and comprehend but has trouble with naming

THE IMPORTANCE OF DEFINING THE APHASIA

The definition of aphasia localizes the _level_ of the nervous system lesion. If aphasia is present, the lesion is usually in the left cerebral cortex. Someone with difficulty using his right hand and a mild aphasia has hemisphere disease, not a brachial plexus lesion.

Aphasia implies dysfunction of middle cerebral artery territory and is often caused by disease of the internal carotid in the neck. Marked stenosis of the internal carotid may be surgically correctable, and if recognized and treated in time a mild or transient aphasia may be prevented from becoming global.

The sudden onset of fluent aphasia without hemiparesis often means an embolus to the posterior branch of the middle cerebral artery. Look for an embolic focus in the heart or in the carotid artery. If the heart is the source, anticoagulation should be considered; if the carotid is the suspected source, angiography is usually performed in search of a surgically remediable lesion. Remember the clinical rule: The sudden onset of aphasia without hemiparesis suggests embolus.

PROGNOSIS OF APHASIA

The prognosis of aphasia in a given patient depends on the location and extent of the lesion. Patients with global aphasia have a poor prognosis and almost never recover completely. Patients with anomic, conduction, and transcortical aphasias have a good prognosis and complete recovery occurs frequently. Broca's and Wernicke's patients have an intermediate prognosis and show a wide range of outcomes. In general, patients with traumatic cases of aphasia do better than those in whom stroke is the cause. The bulk of evidence indicates that speech therapy improves the outcome in aphasia.

NOTE: (1) __Apraxia__ is a disturbance of purposeful movement which cannot be accounted for by elementary motor or sensory impairments or by impaired comprehension or cooperation. It occurs commonly in association with aphasic syndromes and usually involves the "disconnection" of one brain area from another. (2) __Agnosias__ are disorders of recognition which are not accounted for by elementary motor or perceptual disturbances. For example, visual agnosia is a disorder of recognition not accounted for by a primary disorder of vision.   (3) Left posterior parietal disease (Gerstmann's syndrome) includes agraphia, left-right confusion, finger agnosia, and difficulty with calculations.

Disconnection Syndromes

Disconnection syndromes occur when one part of the cortex is disconnected from the other. Examples include: 1) __alexia without agraphia__: patient can write but cannot read - lesion in the left occipital region and adjacent corpus callosum; 2) __Balint's syndrome__: patient has visual inattention and cannot direct gaze to specific points in the visual field despite full extraocular movement - bilateral occipital lesions; 3) __pure word deafness__: patient cannot interpret words or repeat what is said, but can hear and can interpret written language - deep left temporal lobe lesion; 4) __ideomotor apraxia__: patient uses left hand well for all functions except those suggested by verbal commands - lesion in left frontal cortex and adjacent corpus callosum.

REFERENCES

1.   Benson DF: __Aphasia, Alexia and Agraphia__.
     Churchill Livingstone (New York) 1979.
2.   Benson DF, Geschwind N: Aphasia and related
     disturbances, in __Clinical Neurology__, edit. Baker
     and Baker, Harper & Row (New York), Chapter 8, 1982.
3.   Geschwind N: Current concepts: Aphasia. __N Engl J
     Med__ 284:654, 1971.
4.   Holland AL: Treatment for aphasia following stroke.
     __Current Concepts Cerebrovasc Disease__ 14(2):5-8,
     1979.
5.   Kertesz A, McCabe P: Recovery patterns and prognosis
     in aphasia. __Brain__ 100:1, 1977.
6.   Strub RL, Black FW: __The Mental Status Examination
     in Neurology__. F.A. Davis Co., Philadelphia, 1977.

Chapter 5

Stroke

Stroke is one of the most common neurological problems confronting the internist. Some aspects of the treatment of stroke (embolus, thrombosis, hemorrhage) are controversial. A basic approach to the patient with stoke is presented and generally accepted modalities of treatment are outlined.

WHERE IS THE STROKE? WHAT IS THE ANATOMY?

Emboli tend to go peripherally, giving cortical deficits. Intracranial hemorrhage is usually deep, most commonly affecting putamen, thalamus, pons, or cerebellum. Thrombosis produces a wide variety of syndromes; diagnosis is based on history, anatomy of the deficit, and exclusion of embolus and hemorrhage as possibilities. Lacunes (see Chapter 6) may give characteristic anatomic deficits that identify the stroke. In subarachnoid hemorrhage, the neurologic deficit, if any, depends on where the bleeding occurs.

HOW DID THE STROKE DEVELOP?

Emboli usually give maximal deficit at onset and occur most often during waking hours. The deficit may improve within one to two days, sometimes within hours. There usually is no warning. There may be headache and/or focal seizures.

Intracranial hemorrhage also occurs during waking hours, usually in a known hypertensive patient or in a

16

patient with a bleeding tendency (e.g., anticoagulation).
The full deficit is seldom present at onset but develops
gradually over minutes to hours. There is no warning, and
headache, nausea, and vomiting are usually but not
invariably present.

Thrombosis often occurs during sleep or is present
upon arising in the morning. Symptoms and signs usually
progress in a stepwise fashion; it may take hours or days
for the full deficit to develop. The patient often has a
headache and frequently

// A warning is common in
thrombotic strokes //

was warned of the attack -- viz., previous transient
neurologic symptoms or a transient ischemic attack (TIA).
A warning is common in thrombotic strokes and should
always be diligently sought.

1.   TIAs in Carotid Distribution
      . Transient blindness in the eye on the same
        side as a narrowed internal carotid artery
        (amaurosis fugax). Patient may report a
        "shade coming down" over his eye.

      . Transient aphasia.

      . Motor and sensory symptoms in a single
        extemity (upper or lower), or a clumsy
        "bear's paw" hand.

2.   TIAs in Vertebrobasilar Distribution
      . Slurred speech, dizziness, ataxia, syncope,
        dysphagia, numbness around lips or face, double
        vision.

      . Hemiparesis and hemisensory loss do not
        parallel each other in the individual
        limb as in carotid disease. There may be bilateral
        motor or sensory deficits from a single lesion.

Lacunar or small vessel strokes occur abrubtly
or in a stuttering fashion over hours or days. There may
be a warning. Headache is absent.

Subarachnoid hemorrhage occurs abruptly with
severe headache as the cardinal feature, often coming on
during physical exertion.

WHAT ARE THE HISTORICAL CLUES
AND PHYSICAL FINDINGS?

Is There Evidence for Occlusion or Narrowing
of Internal or Common Carotid Artery?

1. Check for (a) decreased or absent pulsation of the carotid in the neck; (b) a bruit over the carotid.

2. Is there an increase in ipsilateral external carotid pulses in the face (superficial temporal, brow, angular) -- representing collateral circulation around an occluded internal carotid? Check for symmetry of these pulses between sides of the face.

3. A Horner's syndrome may be seen ipsilateral to a common carotid occlusion.

4. Patients with hypertension may have less hypertensive change in the fundus on the side of carotid narrowing.

5. Non-invasive techniques to detect carotid stenosis or occlusion include: (a) ophthalmodynamometry (ODN) and ophthalmoplethysmography (OPG) which measure ophthalmic artery pressure (the ophthalmic artery is the first branch of the internal carotid); (b) phonoangiography, which analyzes carotid bruits; (c) Doppler ultrasonography which evaluates periorbital collateral channels; (d) radionucleotide flow scans which detect delayed flow to one hemisphere; and (e) digital subtraction angiography. While cerebral arteriography remains the definitive method for visualizing the carotid circulation, these non-invasive methods are playing an increasingly important role in the detection of cerebrovascular disease and the prevention of stroke.

6. Cholesterol emboli (shiny refractile bodies) may be seen in the retinal arteries on the same side as a diseased carotid.

7. When dealing with stroke in young adults, pursue risk factors such as use of oral contraceptives, possible drug abuse, previously undetected hypertension or mitral valve prolapse.

Large or Small Vessel Disease?

Warning symptoms tend to be stereotyped in small vessel disease and occur over hours to days. In large vessel disease the symptoms frequently vary depending on which territory of the vessel is involved during the warning; symptoms usually precede the stroke by days or weeks, but may occur over a period of months.

Headache is common with large vessel occlusion. Posterior circulation stroke often produces headache over the occiput, and anterior circulation stroke usually produces headache behind the eyes or over the forehead or temples. Headache rarely accompanies small vessel occlusion.

Is There an Embolic Focus?

The heart is the most common source of emboli, though they may arise from a plaque in a diseased carotid artery or aorta. Cardiac factors predisposing to emboli include mural thrombus associated with myocardial infarction (MI), especially anterior MI's or those associated with a hypodynamic left ventricle -- emboli usually occur within ten days but sometimes months after the MI and may be the presenting feature of an MI -- mitral valve disease and atrial fibrillation. Less common cardiac factors include prosthetic or calcified valves, bacterial endocarditis, marantic endocarditis, and atrial myxoma.

NOTE: It is important to realize that there are exceptions to the above rules. Emboli can progress in a stepwise fashion, thrombosis can occur during the day, and hemorrhage may masquerade as thrombosis. Nevertheless, these rules are useful; when combined with other information about the patient, they help guide to the diagnosis.

LABORATORY EXAMINATION

Computerized Assisted Tomography (CAT Scan)
(also see Chapter 27)

The CAT scan is useful in separating hemorrhagic (intracerebral or subarachnoid hemorrhage) from non-hemorrhagic (thrombotic or embolic) stroke. Blood present in a fresh hemorrhage produces an area of increased density, infarction produces an area of decreased density. In addition, the CAT scan may help define the location and size of the abnormality, e.g., vascular territory, superficial or deep location, small or extensive tissue involvement. Specific points include:

1. The CAT scan is positive in virtually all cases of <u>intracerebral hemorrhage (increased density)</u> and often shows inter-hemispheric blood or bleeding into brain parenchyma in subarachnoid hemorrhage. These changes are evident within the first hour after onset of symptoms. With the advent of CAT scanning, many patients with the clinical diagnosis of thrombosis have been found to have intracerebral hemorrhage.

2. The CAT scan is positive in most cases of <u>cerebral infarction (decreased density)</u>, but these changes may only be evident 24 to 48 hours after the onset of symptoms. With contrast enhancement infarcts may mimic tumors on CAT scan, but the enhancement is generally not associated with the significant mass effect that occurs with enhancement of brain tumors. In some instances, a mass effect may be present with infarction, raising the question of a brain tumor; serial scans and clinical observation will clarify the diagnosis.

3. A <u>hemorrhagic infarct</u> secondary to an embolus produces increased density on CAT scan and anti-coagulation should be delayed when hemorrhage is associated with embolic infarction.

4. <u>Brain stem</u> hemorrhage may be visible on CAT scan, brain stem infarction is not.

5. The CAT scan identifies major <u>shifts of intracranial contents</u> which may require cerebral antiswelling agents or even surgical intervention (intracerebral hemorrhage).

6. <u>Subdural hematomas</u> may be recognized on CAT scan by shifts of intracranial contents, partial obliteration of a lateral ventricle or of sulci, and changes in density (depending on the age of the lesion) on the surface of the brain.

7. <u>Brain tumors</u> are identified on CAT scan by characteristic density patterns, contrast enhancement and mass effects.

Lumbar Puncture (LP)

If the cerebrospinal fluid (CSF) is bloody (greater than 1,000 red blood cells) and the pressure is elevated (greater than 200 mm H O), the LP supports hemorrhage. Remember, about 10% of intracerebral hemorrhages show no cells in the CSF, and a normal pressure. All subarachnoid hemorrhages show grossly bloody CSF, usually greater than 25,000 cells.

A lumbar puncture with 50 to 500 red blood cells (RBCs), is suggestive of embolus, though in the majority of emboli the CSF is clear.

No cells are the expected finding in thrombosis and lacunes. Interestingly, white blood cells (WBCs) may sometimes be seen in the CSF after thrombosis or hemorrhage. Large numbers of red cells (10,000-20,000) are occasionally seen after a hemorrhagic infarct secondary to an embolus. An LP (see Chapter 26) is performed when:

. Infection is suspected.

. Subarchnoid hemorrhage is a diagnostic possibility.

. Intracerebral hemorrhage is a diagnostic possibility, a CAT scan (see above) is not readily available, and there are no signs of increased intracranial pressure.

. Before beginning anticoagulation to rule out bleeding, particularly if CAT scan is not available.

. Diagnosis is not clear.

EEG

The EEG may help to localize cortical and sometimes thalamic deficits. It is usually normal in posterior circulation strokes or lacunar (small vessel) disease

// EEG -- usually abnormal with
large vessel disease or emboli //

TABLE 1 CHARACTERISTIC FEATURES OF STROKE

	Embolus	Intra-cerebral hemorrhage	Large vessel thrombosis	Lacune	Subarachnoid hemorrhage
Location	Peripheral (cortical)	Deep (basal ganglia, thalamus, cerebellum)	Variable (depends on vessel)	Pons, internal capsule,	Vessels at junction of the Circle of Willis
Onset	Sudden (maximum deficit at onset)	Sudden (deficit develops over minutes to hours)	Sudden, Gradual, Stepwise, or Stuttering	Sudden, Gradual, Stepwise, or Stuttering	Sudden, Usually few or no focal signs
When	Awake	Awake and active	Asleep or inactive	Asleep or inactive	Awake and active
Warning (TIA)	None	None	Usually	Variable, TIA's may occur	None

22

TABLE 1   CHARACTERISTIC FEATURES OF STROKE (Cont'd.)

	Embolus	Intra-cerebral hemorrhage	Large vessel thrombosis	Lacune	Subarachnoid hemorrhage
Headache	Sometimes	Usually	Sometimes	No	Always (stiff neck)
CAT scan	Decreased density	Increased density	Decreased density	Usually normal	Usually abnormal
LP	Usually clear	Usually bloody	Clear	Clear	Invariably bloody

These characterizations are generally accepted principles regarding stroke; however, remember they are not hard rules, and stroke can present atypically.

and abnormal in anterior circulation large vessel disease or with emboli. It is important to do an EEG if seizure activity is suspected.

Brain Scan

The brain scan usually becomes positive seven to ten days after thrombosis or embolus, and is usually positive earlier in hemorrhage. It is negative in lacunar strokes and may not be positive in thrombotic and embolic strokes. Its role in the diagnosis of cerebrovascular disease has been largely replaced by the CAT scan.

Arteriography

Arteriography is performed (1) to identify surgically correctable lesions (e.g., intracranial aneurysms and arteriovenous malformations, carotid artery stenosis, and ulcerated carotid plaques), (2) to clarify an uncertain diagnosis, and (3) sometimes when anticoagulation is planned to be absolutely certain of the diagnosis. In guiding arteriography it is important to decide clinically whether disease is in the carotid or vertebrobasilar system. Wherever possible, angiography should be done by selective catheterization techniques.

TREATMENT OF STROKE

1. **Anticoagulation** is beneficial in preventing further embolization in patients with cardiac emboli (unless the source is bacterial or marantic endocarditis. Thus, diagnosing an embolus of cardiac origin is crucial. It is important to perform a CAT scan to rule out bleeding before beginning anticoagulation. An LP may be done, but it is less sensitive than a CAT scan in demonstrating intracerebral hemorrhage and carries the risk of spinal hematoma in anticoagulated patients. The timing of anticoagulation after embolism remains controversial. Some physicians anticoagulate immediately, others wait 48 hours; still others wait 10-14 days if the neurologic deficit is massive to avoid converting a pale infarct into a hemorrhagic one. We feel that the weight of evidence favors immediate anticoagulation if hemorrhage has been excluded. Begin with heparin, then switch to warfarin. If the embolus is due to a mural thrombus associated with an MI, anticoagulation is usually continued for six months. If atrial fibrillation and/or rheumatic valvular disease is the cause, long-term anticoagulation is indicated.

2. Most studies on <u>transient ischemic attacks</u> (TIAs) have shown a statistically significant reduction of TIAs and subsequent strokes in patients treated with <u>anticoagulants</u>. There are few bleeding complications when the prothrombin time is well controlled, and when high-risk anticoagulant patients are excluded. It appears there is a beneficial effect of anticoagulants in patients with "stroke in evolution". Many studies did not distinguish those patients with large or small vessel disease, with TIAs in the anterior or posterior circulation, and arteriography was not carried out in all instances. We believe that anticoagulation benefits patients with a severely narrowed but nonoccluded large blood vessel and those who have an ulcerated or irregular plaque that may form the nidus of embolic material. In the latter group, it is not certain whether surgery, antiplatelet agents, or warfarin is the best treatment but most centers favor surgery (endarterectomy) where angiography and endarterectomy can be done with low morbidity and mortality. We feel anticoagulation is not likely to benefit patients with small vessel disease, a completed stroke, or a completely occluded large vessel.

3. At the present time, we favor the Mayo Clinic guidelines (Mayo Clinic Proc. 53:665, 1978) for the management of transient ischemic attacks, which are as follows:

    . The majority of patients with vertebrobasilar TIAs are treated medically.

    . If a skilled surgeon and an experienced angio-grapher are available, patients with typical carotid TIAs who are suitable medical risks should have angiography followed by carotid endarter-ectomy if an appropriate lesion is found.

    . Nonoperated patients with TIAs of less than 2 months' duration are treated with 3 months of warfarin therapy (unless contraindicated) before treatment with aspirin is begun.

    . Nonoperated patients with continuing TIAs of 2 or more months' duration are treated with aspirin unless there has been a recent increase in the frequency, duration, or severity of TIAs. Under

these circumstances, warfarin therapy is advised
for 3 months before aspirin is started. Aspirin
therapy should be continued until the patient has
been free of TIA for one year.

. No treatment is advised for nonoperated patients
  whose last episode of TIA was longer than 12
  months ago.

4. Platelet inhibiting drugs such as aspirin,
   dipyridamole, and sulfinpyrazone have been
   evaluated for treatment of transient ischemic
   attacks and are used by some physicians. The FDA
   has concluded that aspirin is effective in
   reducing the risk of recurrent TIAs in males, but
   not in females. As noted above, we follow the Mayo
   Clinic guidelines for treatment of TIAs. In
   patients who are not candidates for surgery or
   anticoagulation or who have TIAs secondary to
   small vessel disease, we use aspirin in men, and
   aspirin and dipyridamole in women. Clearly, the
   definitive statement on optimal treatment of
   transient ischemic attacks (TIAs) in men and women
   has not yet been achieved.

5. Lowering blood pressure in patients with acute
   stroke may be beneficial when hemorrhage is present
   but can lead to catastrophic results in the face of
   thrombosis or embolism, especially if the blood
   pressure is lowered precipitously. Before acutely
   lowering blood pressure, then, one must be certain of
   the diagnosis.

6. Surgery benefits the following patients:

   . Those with marked unilateral stenosis of one
     carotid who have suffered a mild or transient
     neurologic deficit in that territory
     (endarterectomy).

   . Patients with cerebellar hemorrhage or cerebellar
     infarction with brainstem compression.

   . Nondominant putaminal hemorrhages that form a
     large clot and/or cause herniation. Evacuation
     relieves pressure and prevents brainstem
     compression.

. Although controversial, surgery may benefit patients with asymptomatic, severe carotid stenosis.

<u>Surgery</u> of the carotid artery is not of benefit in complete carotid occlusion or stroke in evolution. Newer techniques, including microsurgical anastomosis of temporal to middle cerebral artery, are being evaluated, particularly for patients with carotid artery occlusion or siphon stenosis who continue to have TIAs.

7. Agents which <u>reduce cerebral edema</u> (see Chapter 24) may benefit patients with large strokes associated with major shifts of intracranial contents during the initial stages of their illness.

8. <u>Cerebral vasodilators</u> (CO_2, papaverine) are of doubtful benefit.

9. Treatment of <u>subarachnoid hemorrhage (SAH)</u> due to aneurysm includes strict bed rest, control of blood pressure, careful medical management, and, whenever possible, surgical ligation or clipping of the aneurysm. Without appropriate treatment approximately 50% of those patients with SAH who survive the first 24 hours, will die within the next two weeks. The clinical condition of the patient, the presence of arterial spasm, and the location of the aneurysm influence surgical intervention. Antifibrinolytic agents (e.g., Amicar) are often given to help prevent rebleeding (they act on systemic fibrinolysins) and some centers use reserpine and kanamycin to decrease vasoactive substances in the brain (dopamine, serotonin) and thus reduce the vasospasm that follows SAH. Nimodipine (a "calcium antagonist") may help reduce cerebral arterial spasm. Vasospasm (narrowing of blood vessels on arteriography plus neurologic symptoms) usually begins 3-14 days after the initial bleed.

10. A comprehensive <u>rehabilitation</u> program which begins in the hospital with physical, occupational, and speech therapy clearly benefits stroke patients. Studies have shown functional gains from such a program that could not be attributed to sponataneous recovery. Likewise, an estimate of the cost/benefit ratio showed that the reduced cost resulting from

returning patients to the family or to independent living more than paid for the cost of providing rehabilitation services.

11. In atypical non-atherosclerotic stroke, the treatment depends on proper diagnosis and then treatment of the underlying disease (e.g., treatment of vasculitis with steroids).

12. Efforts are underway in some communities to prevent stroke by reducing risk factors such as hypertension, cigarette smoking, dietary cholesterol, and by early detection of the stroke-prone patient (e.g., those with TIAs).

REFERENCES

1. Allen GS, et al.: Cerebral arterial spasm - a controlled trial of nimodipine in patients with subarachnoid hemorrhage. N Engl J Med 308:619, 1983.
2. Barnett HJM: Progress towards stroke prevention. Neurology 30:1212, 1980.
3. Barnett HJM: Aspirin in threatened stroke. N Engl J Med 299:53, 1978.
4. Buonano F, Toole JF: Management of patients with established ("computed") cerebral infarction. Stroke 12:7, 1981.
5. Byer JA, Easton JD: Therapy of ischemic cerebrovascular disease. Ann Int Med 93:742, 1980.
6. Cooperative Study: Joint study of extracranial arterial occlusion as a cause of stroke. JAMA 203:153, 159, 1968; 208:509, 1969.
7. Drake CG: Management of cerebral aneurysm. Stroke 12:273, 1981.
8. Easton JD, Sherman DG: Management of cerebral embolism of cardiac origin. Stroke 11(5):433, 1980.
9. Fields WS: Selection of patients with ischemic cerebrovascular disease for arterial surgery. World J Surg 3:147, 1979.
10. Fields WS, et al.: Controlled trial of aspirin in cerebral ischemia. Stroke 8:301, 1977.
11. Genton E, Barnett HJM, Fields WS, et al.: Cerebral ischemia: The role of thrombosis and of antithrombotic therapy. Stroke 8:150, 1977.

12. Ginsberg MD, Greenwood SA, Goldberg HI: Noninvasive diagnosis of extracranial cerebrovascular disease. Neurology 29:623, 1979.
13. Grindal AB, et al.: Cerebral infarction in young adults. Stroke 9:39, 1978.
14. Lee MC, Heaney LM, Jacobson RL, et al.: Cerebrospinal fluid in cerebral hemorrhage and infarction. Stroke 6:638, 1975.
15. Lehmann JF, DeLateur BJ, Fowler RS: Stroke. Does rehabilitation affect outcome? Arhc Phys Med Rehab 56:375, 1975.
16. Millikan CG, McDowell FH: Treatment of progressing stroke. Stroke 12:397, 1981.
17. Mohr JP, Fisher CM, Adams RD: Cerebrovascular diseases. In Harrison's Principles of Internal Medicine. New York, McGraw-Hill.
18. Ruff RL, Dougherty JH: Evaluation of acute cerebral ischemia for anticoagulant therapy: Computed tomography or lumbar puncture. Neurology 31:736, 1981.
19. Silverstein A: Neurologic complications of anticoagulation therapy: a neurologist's view. Arch Int Med 139:217, 1979.
20. Yatsu FM, Mohr J: Anticoagulation therapy for cardiogenic emboli to brain. Neurology 32:274, 1982.

Chapter 6

Selected
Stroke Syndromes

LACUNES

Lacunes are vascular lesions in the brain commonly seen in hypertensive patients. They are tiny areas of thrombotic infarction that become kernel-sized holes pathologically. It is important to recognize lacunar strokes, as they represent small vessel disease and generally require no treatment or further investigation apart from monitoring the patient's medical problems. Control of the patient's blood pressure may help prevent further strokes. Look for these characteristic syndromes:

- <u>Pure motor hemiplegia</u>. Lesion in the pons or internal capsule. Paralysis of face, arm, and leg without sensory loss. If a right hemiplegia, no aphasia. If a left hemiplegia, no parietal lobe findings.

- <u>Pure sensory stroke</u>. Lesion in the thalamus. Sensory loss in face, arm, and leg, with no hemiplegia or other signs.

- <u>Clumsy-hand dysarthria</u>. Lesion in the pons. Slurred speech with clumsiness and mild weakness. of one arm.

- <u>Crural (leg) paresis and ataxia (ataxic hemiparesis)</u>. Lesion in the pons or internal capsule. Ataxia and weakness of one leg.

Pure motor hemiplegia is the easiest to recognize and occurs frequently.

INTRACEREBRAL HEMORRHAGE

*// CAT scan is diagnostic in
intracerebral hemorrhage //*

Bleeding into the <u>cerebellum</u>:

1. Cerebellar hemorrhage is very important to diagnose
    as it can lead to rapid death via brainstem compres-
    sion; treatment is surgical evacuation of the clot.

2. Headache, vomiting, and inability to walk are
    cardinal features.

3. Strength and sensation are usually normal (unless
    brainstem compression occurs).

4. The patient may have trouble looking to the side
    of the lesion (gaze paresis).

5. Nystagmus and limb ataxia are only occasionally
    present.

6. Cerebellar infarction with swelling may mimic
    cerebellar hemorrhage and require surgical
    treatment.

The majority of intracerebral hemorrhages occur in
the <u>putamen</u>. Look for:

. Hemiplegia.

. Striking eye deviation to side of hemorrhage, and
  away from the hemiplegia (Fig. 2).

. Headache, and often a field defect.

. Cortical deficits, which develop as the hemorrhage
  progresses.

Surgical evacuation of the hemorrhage may be useful
in nondominant hemisphere cases, particularly if the
patient's condition deteriorates. Control of blood pressure
is important.

Right putaminal hemorrhage

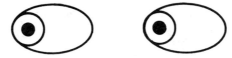

Eyes deviate to the side of the lesion.
Pupils: normal size and reactive.
(seen also with large hemisphere infarcts)

Thalamic hemorrhage

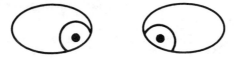

Eyes look down at the nose; vertical gaze is
impaired. Pupils: small and nonreactive.

Pontine hemorrhage

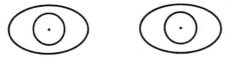

Eyes are midposition with no movement to doll's
eyes maneuver. There may be ocular bobbing.
Pupils: pinpoint, react to light if viewed with a
magnifying glass.

Cerebellar hemorrhage

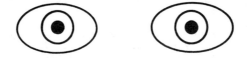

Patient has difficulty looking to the side of the
lesion. There may be skew deviation or a sixth
nerve palsy. Pupils: normal size and reactive.

FIGURE 2   Eye signs of intracerebral hemorrhage.
From Fisher CM: Some neuro-ophthalmological observations.
J Neurol Neurosurg Psychiat 30:383, 1967.

In _thalamic_ hemorrhage, the patient:

. May or may not have hemiplegia.

. Has eyes that look down at his nose, with small
  and nonreactive pupils (Fig. 2).

. Has marked sensory loss.

Supportive treatment is the only modality
available.

Hemorrhage in the _pons_ is usually fatal:

. Patient is comatose with small pinpoint pupils
  (Fig. 2).

. Pupils react to bright light when viewed with a
  magnifying glass.

. Quadriparesis with upgoing toes.

. No horizontal extraocular movements.

SUBARCHNOID HEMORRHAGE

Subarchnoid hemorrhage classically presents with the
sudden onset of severe headache during activity, altered
level of consciousness (at times coma), nuchal rigidity,
and a bloody CSF. Some patients may present with headache
and an altered mental status secondary to bleeding that
occurred a few days prior to hospital admission. There are
usually no focal signs, unless the hemorrhage is into the
substance of brain or if arterial spasm exists. Hemorrhage
into the substance of brain appears as an increased density
on CAT scan; arterial spasm generally produces no changes
on CAT scan. Delayed deterioration in patients with
subarachnoid hemorrhage may be due to hydrocephalus,
seizures, cerebral edema, or vasospasm. The most common
locations for aneurysms are at various arterial junction
points around the circle of Willis at the base of the
brain:

1.   Posterior communicating artery: may have an
      associated third nerve palsy.

2.   Anterior communicating complex: frontal lobe
      dysfunction may be present.

3.   Middle cerebral artery: aphasia or nondominant hemisphere findings.

4.   Less common locations include ophthalmic artery (unilateral blindness), cavernous sinus (ophthalmoplegia), and basilar artery (brainstem signs). Arteriovenous malformations may be found anywhere in the brain, but are most common over the convexities.

THROMBOTIC STROKES

The middle cerebral artery syndrome is seldom due to thrombosis of the middle cerebral artery; it is usually secondary to an occluded carotid in the neck or an embolus to the middle cerebral. Look for:

. Hemiparesis (greater in face and arm than leg)

. Aphasia or nondominant hemisphere findings (depending on the side)

. Cortical sensory loss (greater in face and arm than leg)

. Homonymous hemianopsia

. Conjugate eye deviation (to the side of the hemisphere lesion)

. "Partial" middle cerebral artery syndromes, almost always of embolic origin, may include a) sensorimotor paresis with little aphasia, b) conduction aphasia, c) Wernicke's aphasia without hemiparesis.

In the anterior cerebral artery syndrome look for:

. Paralysis of the lower extremity

. Cortical sensory loss in leg only

. Incontinence

. Grasp and suck reflexes

. Slowness in mentation with perseveration

. No hemianopsia or aphasia

. Left limb apraxia

With occlusion of the <u>internal carotid artery</u> a picture resembling occlusion of the middle cerebral artery occurs. When anterior cerebral territory is included in the area of infarction, clinical features of anterior cerebral occlusion also occur. These patients tend to be stuporous or semicomatose due to the large area of infarction usually present.

The <u>posterior cerebral artery syndrome</u> presents these features:

- Homonymous hemianopsia (often the only finding); the patient may be unaware of the deficit

- Little or no paralysis

- Prominent sensory loss, including to pinprick and touch, may be seen

- No aphasia or nondominant hemisphere dysfunction

- Left posterior cerebral artery syndrome may show ability to write but not read (alexia without agraphia) and inability to name colors

- Recent memory loss may be present (involvement of hippocampus)

Watershed or <u>borderzone infarction syndromes</u> (common after anoxia) include proximal arm weakness with distal sparing and transcortical aphasias (see Chapter 4).

<u>Brainstem syndromes</u> never have cortical deficits or visual field defects. One of the most common brainstem syndromes is the <u>lateral medullary syndrome</u> due to occlusion of the vertebral or posterior inferior cerebellar artery (see Fig. 9, Chapter 28). Look for:

- Ipsilateral to the lesion: facial numbness, limb ataxia, Horner's syndrome (miosis, ptosis, anhydrosis), pain over the eye

- Contralateral to the lesion: pinprick and temperature loss in arm and leg

- Vertigo, nausea, hiccups, hoarseness, difficulty swallowing, and diplopia

If the lesion is typical, treatment is supportive and these patients usually do well. (Beware of aspiration because of swallowing difficulty.)

Most other brainstem strokes are in the pons (see Fig. 10, Chapter 28).

1.   If the lesion is in the medial portion of the pons, there is weakness and an internuclear ophthalmoplegia or gaze palsy with little sensory loss.

2.   If the lesion is in the lateral and tegmental portion of the pons, sensory loss predominates.

3.   Cerebellar signs are present in lateral lesions and are ipsilateral to the lesion.

4.   The level of the pons affected is determined by which cranial nerves are involved. The facial (VII) nerve exits from the lower pons and, if involved there, produces ipsilateral total (upper and lower) facial paralysis. If involved higher, there is contralateral facial paralysis that spares the forehead musculature. The trigeminal (V) nerve exits from the middle of the pons and, if involved at this level, produces ipsilateral loss of corneal reflex and facial sensory loss. The descending tract of the trigeminal (V) nerve runs from midpons to lower medulla, and involvement anywhere in its course results in ipsilateral facial pinprick and temperature loss. In high pontine lesions, pain and sensory loss are contralateral to the lesion in both face and extremities. In brainstem lesions below the high pons, pain and temperature sensations are lost ipsilaterally in the face and contralaterally in the limbs. The cochlear (VIII) nucleus and nerve are in the lower pons and thus ipsilateral deafness and vertigo may accompany pontine lesions.

5.   Midbrain strokes frequently involve the third nerve or nucleus and cerebral peduncle, thus producing ipsilateral pupil dilitation, ptosis, and ophthalmoparesis and contralateral hemiplegia (Weber's syndrome)(See Fig. 11, Chapter 28).

If the deficit in a brainstem stroke is confined to one anatomical area, it generally means that a single branch vessel is involved. If the deficit involves a wider area, the problem may be in the basilar artery itself and catastrophic basilar occlusion may result. Anticoagulation with heparin may prevent the progression from a partial to a complete basilar thrombosis.

NOTE: Rarely, stroke occurs in the spinal cord and presents as paraplegia with urinary retention; a sensory level can usually be found. Vibration and position sense are spared because the etiology is often occlusion of the anterior spinal artery with sparing of the posterior columns. The thoracic cord is most often affected. Treatment is symptomatic and considerable recovery usually occurs.

REFERENCES

1. Castaigne P, Lhermitte F, Gautier JC, et al.: Internal carotid artery occlusion: A study of 61 instances in 50 patients with postmortem data. Brain 93:231, 1970.
2. Currier RD, Giles CL, DeJong RN: Some comments on Wallenberg's Lateral Medullary Syndrome. Neurology 11:778, 1961.
3. Donnan GA, Tress BM, Bladin PF: A prospective study of lacunar infarction using computed tomography. Neurology 32:49, 1982.
4. Hier DB. Davis KR, Richardson EP, et al.: Hypertensive putaminal hemorrhage. Ann Neurol 1:152, 1977.
5. Lehrich JR, Winkler GF, Ojemann RG: Cerebellar infarction with brainstem compression. Arch Neurol 22:490, 1970.
6. Mohr JP: Lacunes. Stroke 13:3, 1982.
7. Mohr JP, Fisher CM, Adams RD: Cerebrovascular diseases. In Harrison's Principles of Internal Medicine. New York, McGraw-Hill, 1983.
8. Pessin MS, Hinton RC, Davis KR, et al.: Mechanism of acute carotid stroke. Ann Neurol 6:245, 1979.
9. Ott KH, Kase CS, Ojemann RG. et al.: Cerebellar hemorrhage. Diagnosis and treatment. Arch Neurol 31:160, 1974.
10. Ropper AH, Davis KR: Lobar cerebral hemorrhages: Acute clinical syndromes in 26 cases. Ann Neurol 8:141, 1979.

11.   Silver JR, Buxton PH: Spinal stroke. Brain
       97:539, 1974.
12.   Walshe TM, Davis KR, Fisher CM: Thalamic hemorrhage:
       A computed tomographic-clinical correlation.
       Neurology 27:217, 1977.

Chapter 7

Transient
Ischemic Attack

The transient ischemic attack (TIA) is an acute
neurologic deficit of vascular origin that clears
completely; it usually lasts minutes to hours, but no more
than 24 hours. In some patients a neurologic deficit
related to focal cerebral ischemia persists for more than
24 hours, but then clears completely (reversible ischemic
neurologic deficit [RIND]). The approach to these
patients is similar to that for the patient with TIAs. A
TIA is important to recognize because it may be a warning
that a more catastrophic and permanent neurologic deficit
is imminent. In some instances, treatment is available
that will help prevent the impending stroke. Between
one-half to two-thirds of people with thrombotic strokes
give a history of a previous TIA, and about one-third of
patients with TIAs will go on to have a stroke within
three years. The symptom complex of TIA represents a
variety of pathophysiologic processes, some better
understood than others. The following points should be
established in the patient with a TIA.

IS THE TIA IN CAROTID OR
VERTEBROBASILAR TERRITORY?

The differential points between these two types of
TIA's -- carotid and vertebrobasilar -- were discussed in
Chapter 5.

TIAs in <u>carotid territory</u> may be associated with
stenosis or ulcerative plaques at the carotid bifurcation
in the neck. When the patient has carotid symptoms,

especially in association with a carotid bruit and/or
decreased carotid pulse, arteriography is usually
performed to define the vascular anatomy and to determine
if he is a candidate for carotid endarterectomy.
Remember, the carotid must be at least 80% narrowed before
the blood flow is significantly decreased. If the TIA is
caused by emboli from an ulcerated plaque, stenosis need
not be present. There are patients who have an occluded
internal carotid with no symptoms at all. Moreover,
patients may have a carotid bruit without stenosis and
stenosis without a bruit. There may be an occlusion with
a palpable pulse or a decreased pulse in a patent vessel.

TIAs in the vertebrobasilar territory are not well
understood. The vertebral arteries and their origins have
a predilection for atheroma development and emboli of
cardiac origin to the vertebrobasilar territory do occur.
Hemodynamic factors may also play a role. Most serious
vertebrobasilar disease is intracranial, where surgery is
not feasible, and the benefit of operation on the
vertebral arteries in the neck is unproven.

In the subclavian steal syndrome the patient has a
narrowed subclavian artery proximal to the origin of the
vertebral artery and the arm "steals" blood from the
basilar artery via the vertebral artery. There may be a
cervical bruit and a difference in blood pressure between
arms. At times of exercise the patient may experience
symptoms of vertebrobasilar insufficiency. In contrast to
other patients with TIAs, those with the subclavian steal
syndrome rarely develop a stroke due to the steal,
although there may be coexistent serious disease in the
carotid arteries.

Vertigo alone is rarely a symptom of vertebrobasilar insufficiency unless other brainstem signs or symptoms
are present. Occasionally, an elderly patient may have
vertebrobasilar symptoms when he turns his head, these
being secondary to mechanical factors in the cervical
region which reduce blood flow.

IS THE HEART
THE SOURCE OF THE TIA?

Emboli from the heart are well-recognized causes of
TIAs in both the carotid and vertebrobasilar systems (more
common in the carotid) and are seen in rheumatic heart

disease, atrial fibrillation, mural thrombus after myocardial infarction, bacterial and marantic endocarditis, atrial myxoma, and with prosthetic valves. Echo cardiography is often helpful in diagnosis, especially in patients with known heart disease.

// Don't confuse Stokes-Adams
attacks with TIA's //

Cardiac arrhythmias may cause TIAs via decreased cardiac output and may require Holter monitoring for identification. Don't confuse Stokes-Adams attacks with a TIA. Stokes-Adams attacks generally do not have focal neurologic signs.

Hypotension may cause focal neurologic symptoms in a patient with compromised cerebral circulation.

TIA: A MIGRAINOUS OR
CONVULSIVE PHENOMENON?

Migraine may be accompanied by transient neurologic deficits (visual disturbances, motor or sensory symptoms) and can usually be identified by the headache that follows the neurologic deficit, the gastrointestinal symptoms, and by the fact that it appears in patients younger than those with cerebrovascular disease. Nevertheless, older people do experience migrainous phenomena, and there may not be prominent headache symptoms. Thus, migraine variants in the elderly pose a difficult diagnostic and therapeutic problem.

Keep in mind that _focal_ _seizures_ may produce transient neurologic symptoms (numbness, leg or arm movement or weakness) which may persist for hours. Obtain an EEG if seizures are suspected. In addition, _chronic_ _subdural hematoma_ and _unruptured cerebral aneurysms_ have been reported to present as recurrent transient neurologic deficits.

Some _systemic factors_ may be associated with or mimic TIAs. Well recognized factors are anemia, polycythemia, thrombocytosis, hyper- and hypoglycemia.

Transient global amnesia (TGA) is a unique syndrome in which, typically, a middle-aged patient suddenly loses recent memory, becomes confused, and asks repeated

questions. The patient appears alert, has no motor or
sensory signs or symptoms and retains "personal identity"
and the ability to answer questions about job, address,
etc. The etiology of this dramatic syndrome is unknown,
but theories include ischemia involving the hippocampal-
fornical system, a seizure phenomenon, or a migraine
variant. Attacks of TGA are often triggered by special
circumstances such as emotional experiences, pain, or
sexual intercourse. Attacks usually last hours and clear
without residual deficit. These patients often have risk
factors for cerebrovascular disease, especially
hypertension. Unless attacks are recurrent, treatment,
except for risk factors, is usually not necessary.

TREATMENT OF THE PATIENT WITH TIA

After a complete work-up (including EKG, auscultation
for bruits, blood pressure check in both arms,
non-invasive tests such as ophthalmoplethysmography, and
sometimes EEG), arteriography may be necessary before
deciding on a mode of treatment. To what extent
arteriography is indicated depends on the neurologist's
and surgeon's evaluations.

Most clinicians believe the endarterectomy is
warranted when there is a unilateral significantly
stenosed or ulcerated carotid in a patient with TIAs in
that vessel's territory.

Many studies on TIAs and anticoagulation show a
statistically significant reduction of TIAs and subsequent
strokes in anticoagulated patients (see Chapter 5 for
discussion of the treatment of TIAs).

A patient is more likely to have a stroke after a few
recent TIAs than after TIAs occurring in the distant past.
There are a large number of TIAs for which no etiology can
be found (e.g., normal cerebral arteriogram and normal
cardiac status); this obviously makes rationale for
treatment difficult. Possible explanations include:

- Some TIA's may be associated with small vessel
  disease not demonstrable on angiography.

- Emboli which result in TIAs may break up as the
  TIA resolves.

REFERENCES

1. Dyken ML: Assessment of the role of anti-platelet aggregating agents in transient ischemic attacks, stroke, and death. Stroke 10:602, 1979.
2. Ennix CL, et al.: Improved results of carotid endarterectomy in patients with symptomatic coronary disease: An analysis of 1,546 consecutive operations. Stroke 10:122, 1979.
3. Fields WS, Lemak NA: Subclavian steal: A review of 168 cases. JAMA 222:1139, 1972.
4. Fisher CM: Migraine accompaniments versus arteriosclerotic ischemia. Trans Am Neurol Assoc 93:211, 1968.
5. Fisher CM: Transient global amnesia. Arch Neurol 39:605, 1982.
6. Jonas S, Klein I, Dimant J: Importance of Holter monitoring in patients with periodic cerebral symptoms. Ann Neurol 1:470, 1977.
7. Marshall J, Meadows S: The natural history of amaurosis fugax. Brain 91:419, 1968.
8. Millikan CH, McDowell FH: Treatment of transient ischemic attacks. Stroke 9:299, 1978.
9. Olsson JE, et al.: Anti-coagulant vs anti-platelet therapy as prophylaxis against cerebral infarction in transient ischemic attacks. Stroke 11:4, 1980.
10. Sandok B, Furlan A, Whisnant J, et al.: Guidelines for the management of transient ischemic attacks. Mayo Clin Proc 53:665, 1978.
11. Shuping JR: Transient global amnesia. Ann Neurol 7:281, 1980.
12. Stewart RM, Samson D, Diehl, et al.: Unruptured cerebral aneurysms presenting as recurrent transient neurologic deficits. Neurology 30:47, 1980.
13. Toole JF, Yuson CP: Transient ischemic attacks with normal arteriograms: Serious or benign prognosis? Ann Neurol 1:100, 1977.
14. Toole JF, Yuson CP, Janeway R, et al.: Transient ischemic attacks: A prospective study of 225 patients. Neurology 28:746, 1978.
15. Welsh JE, Tyson GW, Winn HR, et al.: Chronic subdural hematoma presenting as transient neurologic deficits. Stroke 10:564, 1979.

Chapter 8

Coma

Proper evaluation of the comatose patient usually involves obtaining a history from family and friends, a rapid directed physical and neurological examination, and obtaining certain laboratory studies, while the patient's airway and vital signs are protected. These various parts of the evaluation are often proceeding simultaneously, e.g., one member of the medical team securing the airway, while another is talking to the family. An attempt is made to delineate the cause of coma in hopes of finding a treatable process. Treatable causes of coma include metabolic derangements, ingestions, and at times supratentorial processes in the brain (e.g., epidural hematoma). Anatomically, coma implies bilateral hemisphere dysfunction, either structural, drug induced, or metabolic, unilateral hemisphere disease with compression of brainstem (e.g., epidural hematoma), or brainstem dysfunction (e.g., pontine hemorrhage or compression from a posterior fossa mass). If certain basic points are established when examining the comatose patient, the extent of structural CNS derangement and the cause usually can be determined.

HISTORY

1. Learn from family or friends whether the patient has a pre-existing condition that might explain his coma. Is he a diabetic? Is he a drug addict? Does he take sleeping pills? Has he been depressed? Has there been recent head trauma?

2. If a pre-existing medical condition exists, is there a factor that may have exacerbated it and

precipitated the coma? E.g., chronic liver disease and GI bleeding; uremia and infection; a seizure disorder and failure to take anticonvulsant medication.

EXAMINATION

OBSERVE THE PATIENT CAREFULLY

1.   Is there decorticate posturing (arm flexion with leg extension), implying hemisphere or diencephalon dysfunction which may be due to destructive lesions or be secondary to a metabolic derangement.

2.   Is there decerebrate posturing (extension of legs and arms), implying dysfunction of midbrain or upper pons on a structural or metabolic basis.

3.   Is the patient yawning, swallowing, or licking his lips? If so, coma cannot be very deep and brainstem function is probably intact.

4.   Are there repetitive, multifocal myoclonic jerks or multifocal seizures. These are characteristic of metabolic encephalopathies such as hypoxia or uremia.

WHAT IS THE RESPIRATORY PATTERN?

Cheyne-Stokes respiration (a crescendo-decrescendo breathing pattern with apneic pauses in between) implies bilateral hemisphere dysfunction with an intact brainstem and may be the first sign of transtentorial herniation; it also accompanies metabolic disorders and congestive heart failure.

Central neurogenic hyperventilation (rapid deep breathing) usually indicates damage to the brainstem tegmentum between midbrain and pons.

Apneustic breathing consists of a prolonged inspiratory cramp followed by an expiratory pause and is usually seen in pontine infarction.

Ataxic (irregular or agonal) breathing is usually a pre-terminal event signifying disruption of medullary centers.

Remember, significant damage to the brainstem is rarely accompanied by a normal breathing pattern.

Coma with hyperventilation frequently signifies
a metabolic derangement:

. Metabolic acidosis: diabetes, uremia, lactic
  acidosis, poisoning

. Respiratory alkalosis: salicylates, hepatic
  failure

Coma with hypoventilation frequently implies
generalized CNS depression secondary to a drug overdose
and occurs in patients with chronic pulmonary disease
and CO retention.

DOES THE PATIENT RESPOND TO
EXTERNAL STIMULI?

1.   Apply a noxious stimulus to determine whether the
     patient is unresponsive. Noxious stimuli may
     elicit decorticate or decerebrate posturing and
     thus give a clue to the level of brain damage or
     dysfunction.

2.   Test for voluntary response -- e.g., let patient's
     hand fall toward his face and see if he resists (a
     check for malingering).

3.   Check for a response of the limbs to pain: Is there
     a low level reflex such as flexion, extension, or
     adduction? Abduction of shoulder or hip usually
     indicates a higher level (cortical) response. With-
     drawal implies purposeful or voluntary behavior.

EXAMINE THE PUPILS CAREFULLY

Note the size, equality and light reaction of the
pupils.

1.   A metabolic (not structural) lesion is usually
     present if the comatose patient has no response to
     external stimuli, absent doll's eyes and corneal
     reflexes, and yet preserved pupillary responses.
     Such cases are often secondary to barbiturate
     ingestion.

2.   Gluthethimide (Doriden) ingestion and atropine or
     scopolamine poisoning give large unreactive pupils

which give the false impression of a structural
lesion.

3. Normal sized, reactive pupils imply an intact
    midbrain. Midbrain damage usually produces dilated
    pupils which do not react to light but may
    fluctuate in size.

4. Pontine damage produces pinpoint pupils which do
    react to bright light when viewed with a magnifying
    glass. Heroin and pilocarpine also produce
    pinpoint pupils.

5. A unilaterally fixed, dilated pupil is seen with
    damage to the third nerve, and often is a valuable
    early sign of temporal lobe (uncal) herniation from
    a supratentorial lesion (see Chapter 24).

CHECK FOR CORNEAL
REFLEXES AND DOLL'S EYES

Absence of corneal reflexes and doll's eyes usually
means pontine damage or dysfunction. If there is no
doll's eye response, use ice water irrigation, a strong
stimulus of the oculovestibular reflex pathway (be sure
there is no wax in the ears); tonically deviated eyes to
the side of the irrigation, a normal response, signifies
that some brainstem function is intact. Absence of the
oculovestibular response implies severe depression of
brainstem function.

MOTOR SYSTEM EXAMINATION IS IMPORTANT

Hyperreflexia and upgoing toes or hemiplegia
usually mean a structural CNS lesion is the cause of
coma. Some exceptions are hepatic coma, hypoglycemia,
and uremia, which may be associated with focal signs or
hyperreflexia. Nonetheless, these should be quickly
diagnosed by laboratory studies. Hyporeflexia and
downgoing toes with no hemiplegia generally means there
is no structural CNS lesion, and supports drug ingestion
or other metabolic cause.

OTHER PHYSICAL FINDINGS

Careful physical examination may detect other clues to
the cause of coma, for example, signs of head trauma in

epidural hematoma, barrel chest in pulmonary failure, hepatomegaly in hepatic coma, feeble pulse and hypotension in cardiogenic shock, and stiff neck in meningitis or subarchnoid hemorrhage. There may be cyanosis with hypoxia or "cherry red" appearance in carbon monoxide poisoning. Hypothermia may be associated with barbiturate or ethanol ingestion, while hyperthermia may occur in heat stroke.

LABORATORY STUDIES

Laboratory studies must be carried out to exclude metabolic causes of coma such as hypoglycemia, hypercapnia, hypercalcemia, uremia, hepatic failure, electrolyte disturbance, or toxin ingestion. When clinically appropriate, a CAT scan is indicated to rule out intracranial hemorrhage (subdural, epidural, or intracerebral). A lumbar puncture may be needed to detect infection or subarachnoid hemorrhage, although one must be certain there is no shift of midline structures prior to the lumbar puncture.

// Hypoglycemia is one of
the most treatable causes
of coma //

Remember: Hypoglycemia is one of the most treatable causes of coma. After drawing a blood glucose, give all comatose patients 50gm glucose intravenously. If there is a possibility of malnutrition, give 100mg of thiamine concurrently to prevent Wernicke's encephalopathy. Naloxone (0.4mg-0.8mg) should be given intravenously if narcotic overdosage is a possibility. Other therapeutic measures, such as treatment of increased intracranial pressure or gastric lavage after ingestions may be required.

Note: A discussion of the approach to the patient who is "brain dead" or who is thought to be in "irreversible coma" is beyond the scope of this manual. Principles found useful for house officers when approaching the latter problems include: a) obtaining appropriate consultations and tests (e.g., EEG) before major therapeutic decisions are made; b) meticulous attention to good communication between all members of the health care team and with family members; c) identification of one physician (usually the admitting physician or primary treating physician) who assumes the primary responsibility for collating the clinical information, consulting with the family, and making the major therapeutic decisions.

REFERENCES

1. Caronna JJ, Simon RP: The comatose patient: A diagnostic approach and treatment. Int Anesthiol Clin 17:3, 1979.
2. Fisher CM: The neurological examination of the comatose patient. Acta Neurol Scand 45(suppl 36): 1:56, 1969.
3. Levy et al.: Prognosis in non-traumatic coma. Ann Int Med 94:293, 1981.
4. Plum F, Posner J: Diagnosis of Stupor and Coma 3rd Ed., Philadelphia, F.A. Davis Company, 1980.

Chapter 9

Headache

Critical to the evaluation of the patient with headache is obtaining a careful history.

CHARACTER OF HEADACHE PAIN

Migraine headaches are periodic, throbbing, severe, frequently unilateral, and often over the eye(s). Photophobia and sensitivity to sound are common, as are nausea and vomiting.

Tension headaches tend to be diffuse, steady, occipital or frontal, and "bandlike".

Headaches associated with increased intracranial pressure or tumor are usually not excruciating like migraine.

Cluster headaches are very painful, knifelike, unilateral, and over the eye.

HOW LONG HAS THE HEADACHE BEEN PRESENT?

Migraine usually starts during teenage years (although it may begin at any age), decreases during the 30's and 40's, and may be exacerbated or relieved during menstruation, pregnancy, or around menopause. There is frequently a family history of migraine or of motion sickness as a child.

Cluster headaches are usually seen in patients 20
to 60 years old. The headaches come in clusters, last
weeks to months, and then subside. Males are more often
affected than females.

Tension headaches are usually seen after age 10,
are most prominent at times of stress and at the end of
the day and usually do not occur in a cyclic pattern.

Headache that slowly increases in intensity and
frequency, does not fit the classic pattern of migraine,
tension, or cluster, and appears in someone who has
never had headaches before, is highly suspicious of
tumor or raised intracranial pressure.

IS THERE A VISUAL OR OTHER PRODROME?

// Migraine may be
classic or common //

Migraine may either be classic (preceded by
visual or other prodrome) or common (no prodrome). The
latter has the same character as classic migraine, but
often develops with no warning or builds up slowly.

Classic migraine usually begins with a visual
prodrome such as flashing lights, blind spots, or hemianopsia. Headache begins when the visual prodrome is over
or subsiding. Other prodromal symptoms may occur with one
symptom leading to another -- e.g., hemianopsia to
difficulty talking, to tingling of face or extremities, to
actual hemiparesis ("hemiplegic migraine"). Sensory
symptoms that spread slowly along an extremity frequently
occur ("marching symptoms"). Classic migraine often has
"positive" symptoms followed by "negative" ones -- e.g.,
flashing lights followed by darkness, tingling followed by
numbness.

Nausea and vomiting are prominent features of
migraine -- thus the designation "sick headaches". The
gastrointestinal disturbance usually occurs after the
headache has been established. Scalp tenderness is also
characteristic.

Eye tearing, facial flushing, stuffy or runny nose
are autonomic phenomena associated with cluster headache
and occur ipsilateral to the headache.

WHEN DO THE HEADACHES OCCUR?

Tension headaches usually appear toward the end of the day.

Migraine may occur at any time, including times of stress, or may awaken the patient from sleep. It may begin during a "relaxed time" -- e.g., on a weekend or vacation, or when a stressful period has ended. Migraine may be associated with menstrual periods or brought on by hunger, (skipped meals), alcohol ingestion, eating chocolate, or at high altitudes. Birth control pills, hyperlipidemia, and hypertension may exacerbate migraine.

Cluster headaches may have the unique feature of occurring at the same time every day. Patients can "set their watches" by the headaches. Cluster headaches, like migraine, may be strong enough to wake a patient and are often precipitated by alcohol.

WHAT FACTORS MAKE THE HEADACHE
BETTER OR WORSE?

Migraine, once established, usually is relieved by sleep and often improves after vomiting.

Sleep has no effect on cluster headache.

Tension headaches are often relieved by relaxation techniques or by massaging the back of the neck.

Headache caused by tumor is often made worse by coughing or by straining during a bowel movement (also seen in migraine) and may be at its worst when the patient arises in the morning.

DOES MEDICATION AFFECT THE HEADACHE?

Tension headaches usually respond to aspirin or acetaminophen.

Ergot given early in the course of migraine often prevents or alleviates the headache; some believe this is diagnostic of migraine.

Cluster headaches are generally not helped by medication once the headache appears.

HOW LONG DOES THE HEADACHE LAST?

Cluster headache lasts minutes to a few hours.

Migraine usually lasts hours to a full day, occasionally longer. Tension headache may become superimposed, prolonging the headache episode ("mixed headache").

Tension headaches usually last hours, but can last days.

IS DEPRESSION A FACTOR?

Depression and anxiety are frequently significant factors. Be certain to understand the patient's life style, personality, etc. This is especially important with a patient who has had headaches "every day" for a prolonged period of time. Explore such issues as adjustment to school or job, domestic strife, illness at home, or recent death.

EXAMINATION OF THE PATIENT WITH HEADACHE

Examination sometimes offers clues to the type of headache or to the presence of organic processes, especially if the patient is symptomatic during the exam.

1. Look carefully for focal signs indicative of tumor or other structural lesion (be sure to visualize the fundi).

2. Check for signs of __autonomic dysfunction__ during the headache if cluster is suspected -- e.g., miotic pupil, ptosis, red eye, unilateral nasal congestion.

3. Note "sweaty" hands and feet or scalp tenderness (migraine).

4. If the patient develops a stiff neck during the "worst headache of my life", suspect subarachnoid hemorrhage.

5. Patients with __arteriovenous malformations__ may present with migraine; be suspicious if migraine attacks are __always__ on the same side. Listen for bruits over the skull or eyes. Migraine which has occurred on either side is usually benign.

6. Headache over the eye in an older person (50 to 70
    years of age) may be due to temporal arteritis.
    Check for a tender temporal artery; the sedimentation
    rate should be elevated. Remember that temporal
    arteritis can lead to blindness, which can be
    prevented by steroids.

7. Note hypertension, which may exacerbate migraine or
    tension headaches, particularly if the hypertension
    is labile.

            // Temporal arteritis and glaucoma
               may present as headache in the
               elderly and lead to blindness //

8. Glaucoma is a cause of headache in the elderly;
    headache, eye pain, and vomiting are common. Pal-
    pate the globe and perform tonometry if glaucoma
    is suspected; treatment with pilocarpine or eye
    surgery may prevent blindness -- thus early diagnosis
    is crucial.

                   TREATMENT TIPS

                     Migraine

            Treatment of the Acute Headache

1. Aspirin or acetaminophen: May help but usually has
    been tried by the patient by the time he comes to the
    doctor.

2. Fiorinal: Is often of benefit but may be habit
    forming.

3. Ergot (various preparations are listed under
    ergotamine tartrate in the PDR): Effective in
    prevention or amelioration of headache if given
    during the prodrome. In some patients, rectal or
    sublingual preparations may be more effective than
    oral administration. Once the headache is
    established, strong analgesia and/or medication to
    induce sleep may be needed. Ergot derivatives are
    contraindicated in hemiplegic migraine and in
    patients with known coronary vasospasm.

Prophylactic Medication

1. <u>Propranolol</u> is useful for migraine prophylaxis;
   most use it before trying methysergide (20 to 40 mg
   q.i.d.). Use with great caution in patients with
   asthma, diabetes, and heart disease.

2. <u>Amitriptyline</u> is useful for migraine prophylaxis.
   Begin with 25-50 mg at bedtime; 100-200 mg at bedtime
   may be needed before an effect is seen.

3. <u>Methysergide</u> (Sansert): Given prophylactically to
   those with frequent incapacitating migraine who have
   not responded to other medication. It is prescribed
   daily but not for more than five months at a time;
   the latter precaution minimizes complications such as
   retroperitoneal fibrosis. It may be restarted after
   a one-month hiatus.

4. <u>Prophylactic phenobarbital</u> or <u>phenytoin</u>:
   Phenobarbital is useful in juvenile migraine. Either
   may be useful in adults; phenytoin may be particularly useful in patients with paroxysmal EEG
   patterns.

5. <u>Diuretics</u>: Helpful if the migraine appears to come
   in association with menstruation. Give three to five
   days before the menstrual period starts (e.g.,
   acetazolamide 250 mg t.i.d.).

6. <u>Antihistamines</u> may be of benefit in some patients
   with migraine, especially when associated with nasal
   congestion. Cyproheptadine (Periactin) has been
   found particularly useful in juvenile migraine.

7. Avoid factors which precipitate migraine, e.g.,
   alcohol, skipped meals, birth control pills, food
   containing tyramine or monosodium glutamate. Many
   patients benefit from regular daily exercise.

8. Non-steroid anti-inflammatory medications, such as
   indomethacin, can provide relief for some patients.
   They may be of particular benefit if given
   prophylactically to patients with exertional
   headache.

Cluster Headaches

1. Cluster headache is often quite refractory to treatment, and medication is of little help once the headache is established.

2. To prevent headache once the cluster series has begun, ergot at bedtime or every 12 hours (suppository or intramuscularly), methysergide, cyproheptadine (Periactin), propranolol, chlorpromazine, or prednisone have been found useful.

3. In chronic cluster headache, indomethacin and lithium have been shown to be effective.

Tension Headache

. Aspirin, Fiorinal, acetaminophen

. Narcotics should not be given for tension headache

. Tranquilizers

. Neck massage and heat

. Relaxation techniques

Headache Associated with Depression

Antidepressants may relieve headache in certain instances; psychotherapy may be necessary.

REFERENCES

1. Caviness VS, O'Brien P: Current concepts: Headache. N Engl J Med 302:446, 1980.
2. Couch JR, Ziegler DK, Hassanein R: Amitriptyline in the prophylaxis of migraine. Neurology 26:121, 1976.
3. Dalessio DJ: Migraine, platelets, and headache prophylaxis. JAMA 239:52, 1978.
4. Diamond S: Symposium on headache: Its diagnosis and management. Headache 19:113, 1979.
5. Diamond S, Medina JL: Double blind study of propranolol for migraine prophylaxis. Headache 16:24, 1976.

6. Editorial: Treatment of migraine. _Lancet_ 1:1338, 1982.

7. Graham JR: Seven common headache profiles. _Neurology_ 13:16, Appendix, 1963.

8. Mathew NT: Prophylaxis of migraine and mixed headache. A randomized controlled study. _Headache_ 21:105, 1981.

9. Wolff H: _Headache and Other Head Pain_, ed 3. New York, Oxford University Press Inc., 1972.

10. Saper JR: Migraine. _J Amer Med Assoc_ 239:2380–2383, 2480–2484, 1978.

Chapter 10

Dementia

Dementia is a loss of intellectual ability that interferes with a person's ability to function in his/her occupation or social situation.

The goal of the physician is to characterize the patient's dementia in search of a treatable cause.

WHAT IS THE NATURE OF THE DEMENTIA?

Obtain a Careful History
from the Family

1. When did difficulties first begin (very important) and how rapidly have they progressed -- e.g., did minor problems occur at work?

2. Has the patient been ataxic, incontinent?

3. Is there a history of getting lost?

4. Has there been a misuse of words?

5. Has the patient become more sloppy in habits or dress?

6. Is the patient friendly or has he become angry and belligerent with the onset of mental difficulties? Has there been a personality change?

7. Has there been toxin exposure (e.g., at work), alcohol, or drug abuse?

8. Is there a history of head trauma before difficulties began? Does the patient complain of headache?

9. Does the patient have an underlying medical illness?

Define the Mental Status

1. Check the **state of consciousness**. If the patient is not fully awake, one should suspect a metabolic disorder or a space-occupying lesion. Clues that the process may be delirium rather than dementia include inattention, fluctuating symptoms, disturbances in sleep, prominent perceptual abnormalities, and increased autonomic activity.

2. Check for **orientation** to place, person, and time.

3. Is the patient **aphasic** (see Chapter 4)? Can he read a newspaper and write to dictation? If so, does he make errors?

4. **New memory**: Can the patient recall three or four unrelated objects after five minutes? Can he remember money placed under his pillow, in his pajama pocket? What is his knowledge of recent current events?

5. **Old memory**: Can he give correct information about events which occurred some years ago (e.g., naming of presidents)?

6. **Calculation**: Give a simple problem -- e.g., six rolls cost 12¢ each; if you give the baker $1.00, how much change would you receive?

7. **Abstraction**: How are a ball and orange alike? What do a bath tub and the ocean have in common?

8. **Judgment**: What would he do if he spotted a fire in a theater; if he found a stamped, addressed envelope in the street?

9. **Pictures**: How well can the patient interpret a picture in a magazine? Does he focus on one tiny part; is he unable to integrate it (visual agnosia)? Can the patient draw or copy designs?

10. What is the patient's **mood** and **mental content**? Is he sad or inappropriately cheerful? Is he fearful

or paranoid? Is he active or apathetic, personally neat or sloppy? Is his affect labile?

Perform Careful General and Neurologic Examinations

1. General examination: Is there evidence of liver, kidney, lung, heart, or thyroid disease?

2. Are there focal signs, such as a field defect or aphasia?

3. Check for pathologic reflexes (e.g., Babinski, suck, snout, grasp).

4. Test for smell. Make certain the patient can hear.

5. Check blood pressure and for evidence of arrhythmia.

DO THE HISTORY AND PHYSICAL SUGGEST A TREATABLE CAUSE?

Is There a Tumor?

1. Tumors presenting silently as dementia are often in the frontal lobe. Frontal lobe reflexes (suck, snout, grasp) may be present, and there is a "slowness" in carrying out tasks. Smell may be impaired. Tumors occurring in other areas usually give focal signs.

2. Tumors obstructing the third or fourth ventricle may cause hydrocephalus and subsequent dementia, often with few focal signs.

3. Memory difficulties or language problems are not common early features of brain tumors.

4. The patient with dementia secondary to brain tumor usually presents within 6 to 12 months of the onset of symptoms. (See Chapter 20 for signs and symptoms of brain tumor.)

5. A normal CAT scan, EEG and spinal fluid pressure and protein (perform LP after CAT scan) are sufficient to rule out tumor.

Normal Pressure Hydrocephalus (NPH)

1. Check for memory deficits, ataxia of gait, and
    incontinence. Lower extremity spasticity and upgoing
    toes are frequent findings. The pathophysiology of
    NPH is not well understood, but involves inadequate
    absorption of CSF over the cerebral hemispheres
    leading to hydrocephalus.

    > // A demented patient with a normal gait
    >   does not have NPH //

2. Deterioration over 6 to 12 months is usual.

3. NPH may follow subarachnoid hemorrhage, meningitis,
    or head trauma, but is often of unknown etiology.

4. If NPH is a serious consideration, CAT scan and
    radionucleotide cisternography* are indicated. The
    patients who are most likely to benefit from a shunt
    procedure are those with a "characteristic" clinical
    history, a short history of deterioration (6-12
    months), and abnormal studies.

Subdural Hematoma

1. Look for drowsiness in an elderly patient with a
    recent personality change. Headache is a very
    important feature and is usually, although not
    invariably present.

2. Mental changes usually occur over days to weeks, and
    sometimes months.

3. There need not be a history of head trauma.

4. Screen for subdural hematoma by performing a CAT or
    brain scan, and EEG. If headache and depressed
    consciousness are prominent and a history of head
    trauma is present, one may perform arteriography (the
    definitive study) even if the CAT scan is negative.

* Radioactive material injected via LP goes into and stays
  in the lateral ventricles rather than over the cerebral
  hemispheres. CAT scan reveals hydrocephalus with normal
  sulci.

5. Bilateral subdural hematoma may appear on CAT scan
    only as bilateral obliteration of cortical sulci,
    ventricular compression may not be evident. The
    diagnosis is confirmed by technetium brain scan or
    arteriography.

6. If one suspects subdural hematoma clinically, do not
    perform a lumbar puncture -- it is not diagnostic and
    may be harmful. (The CSF in patients with subdural
    hematoma may show xanthochromia and elevated protein,
    but is normal in about half of proven cases.)

Vitamin B$_{12}$ Deficiency

1. Onset may be insidious over months to years.

2. Although the patient usually has a megaloblastic
    anemia, he may have a normal blood smear, bone
    marrow, and neurologic examination except for the
    dementia.

3. The EEG is usually abnormal and improves after
    vitamin B$_{12}$ is given.

4. A serum vitamin B$_{12}$ assay is usually a sufficient
    screening test provided that the patient has not been
    recently started on vitamins. However, the B$_{12}$ level
    may be normal in some cases of combined system
    disease and therefore a B$_{12}$ bioassay or Shilling test
    may be necessary for diagnosis.

5. Folate deficiency may produce dementia. Patients who
    have pernicious anemia treated with folate improve
    hematologically but progress neurologically.

6. Look for associated paresthesias and posterior and
    lateral column spinal cord signs (combined system
    disease - see Chapter 18).

Liver Disease

1. Hepatic dysfunction often presents with defects in
    memory, abstracting ability, and attentiveness.

2. Mental changes may occur, even though underlying
    liver disease (such as jaundice) is not apparent.

3. Note somnolence, generalized hyperreflexia,

asterixis, myoclonus, and hyperventilation (with respiratory alkalosis).

4. Obtain liver function studies, including an arterial blood ammonia level.

5. Check ceruloplasmin and 24-hour urinary copper levels to rule out Wilson's disease.

Depression

Remember, depression may present as dementia, and is often termed "pseudodementia". Distinguishing features of pseudodementia include:

1. History of a previous psychiatric disorder is common.

2. Onset usually can be dated and symptoms are usually of brief duration.

3. Patients complain of cognitive loss, yet make little effort to perform even simple tasks; they communicate a strong sense of distress, and give frequent "don't know" answers.

4. Associated features of depression may be present, including social withdrawal, ruminations of guilt, anorexia, weight loss, insomnia, and episodes of crying.

Note:

a. Depression may cause pseudodementia by exacerbating a mild organic dementia.

b. Sometimes a trial of antidepressant medication may be necessary to exclude depression as a contributing factor.

Other Treatable Causes

Check for syphilis (serologic tests of blood and spinal fluid should be positive), fungal meningitis (CSF pleocytosis and decreased glucose), toxin (metals) or bromide poisoning, uremia, myxedema, Cushing's disease, thiamine deficiency, carbon monoxide poisoning, congestive heart failure, drugs such as barbiturates, chronic hypoxia, untreated hypertension, hypercalcemia, carcinoma

of the lung and subacute bacterial endocarditis.   All may
include dementia in their clinical picture.

IS THERE A NONTREATABLE CAUSE?

Alzheimer's Disease
(Presenile Dementia)

1.   When the onset of the dementia is between the ages of
      50 to 65 years it is called presenile dementia.   The
      same disorder (identical pathologically) occurring
      after 65 is the most common cause of senile dementia.

2.   Progression is slow over a period of years.

3.   Look for memory problems, a tendency to get lost, and
      language difficulties.

4.   There are usually no neurologic signs apart from the
      dementia; toes are usually downgoing, and the patient
      is generally sociable and neat in the early stages.
      Later, personality change is frequent and there may
      be visual agnosia (the ability to see parts of but
      not recognize objects).

5.   Pick's disease resembles Alzheimer's clinically but
      is very rare.   Pathologically it affects frontal and
      temporal lobes more than parietal lobes.

6.   CAT scan may or may not show ventricular dilatation
      and cortical atrophy.   EEG shows slowing and
      irregularity of background rhythms.

Arteriosclerosis
(Multiple Strokes)

1.   Arterioslcerotic dementia does not mean "getting
      old"; the term should be reserved for patients with
      multiple vascular infarcts of the brain.

2.   Look for bilateral pyramidal signs, including upgoing
      toes and a history suggesting previous small focal
      lesions.

3.   Note pseudobulbar signs: emotional lability with
      easy crying and laughing, increased jaw jerk and gag,
      dysarthria, and dysphagia.

4. This type of dementia occurs predominantly in inadequately treated hypertensives and is therefore potentially preventable.

Creutzfeldt-Jacob Disease

1. The interval between onset and death is usually months.

2. In addition to dementia, patients have upper motor neuron signs, myoclonus, basal ganglia signs, startle to noise and bright lights, and characteristic EEG changes (paroxysmal high voltage bursts).

3. This disease is caused by an as yet unidentified transmissible agent.

Huntington's Chorea

1. Huntington's Chorea presents as insidious intellectual deterioration in association with chorea. Dementia, personality and emotional disorder may precede the chorea. Inheritance is autosomal dominant, family history is usually positive, but must be diligently explored.

LABORATORY WORK-UP

A basic screen for dementia should include: CBC, urinalysis, electrolytes, sedimentation rate, vitamin B_{12} and folate levels, liver function tests, calcium, BUN, thyroid function tests, serological tests for syphilis, drug levels (where appropriate), EKG, chest X-ray, EEG, CAT scan, LP (if there is no evidence of a mass on the previous studies), and psychological testing (where appropriate).

With a careful history and physical examination and the preceding studies the etiology of dementia should be clear in the vast majority of cases. If the diagnosis remains uncertain, other studies, such as arteriography or brain biopsy, are sometimes necessary. The extent of the work-up depends on the patient's age and previous level of function.

REFERENCES

1. Barrett RE: Dementia in adults. Med Clinic North Am 56:1405, 1972.

2. Dunea G, Mahurkar SD, Mamdani BV. Smith EC: Role of
    aluminum in dialysis dementia. __Ann Int Med__ 88:502,
    1978.
3. Freeman FR: Evaluation of patients with progressive
    intellectual deterioration. __Arch Neurol__ 33:658,
    1976.
4. McEvoy JP: Organic brain syndromes. A review. __Ann__
    __Int Med__ 95:212, 1981.
5. McKissock W: Subdural hematoma: A review of 389
    cases. __Lancet__ 1:367, 1960.
6. Stuteville P, Welch K: Subdural hematoma in the
    elderly person. __JAMA__ 168:1455, 1958.
7. Terry RD: Dementia. A brief and selected review.
    __Arch Neurol__ 33:1, 1976.
8. Terry RD, Davies P: Dementia of the Alzheimer type.
    __Ann Rev Neurosci__ 3:77, 1980.
9. Wells CE: __Dementia.__ 3rd ed., Philadelphia, F.A.
    Davis Company, 1980.

Chapter 11

Seizures

Seizures reflect a disorder of the nervous system due to a sudden, excessive, disorderly discharge of brain neurons.

TYPE OF SEIZURES

Seizures are categorized into two major groups, depending on the source: Focal (partial) seizures and generalized (centrencephalic) seizures. In focal seizures (Fig. 3A) the initial discharge comes from a focal unilateral area of the brain: temporal lobe, frontal lobe, motor strip, etc. Thus, a patient whose seizure begins with his right hand shaking or with an aura of smelling "burned candy" has a focal seizure disorder attributable to a lesion in the frontal or temporal lobe, respectively.

Remember, a seizure can begin focally and then generalize (Fig. 3B); this may happen so quickly that it is impossible to see the focality clinically, and the patient can recall no aura. Nonetheless, the EEG usually shows the focality. Focal seizure disorders are usually secondary to local pathology -- e.g., trauma, tumor, vascular lesions, and congenital abnormalities.

In primary generalized seizures (Fig. 3C) the discharge arises from deep midline structures in the brainstem or thalamus. There is no aura and there are no focal features during the seizure. Examples of primary generalized seizure disorders are petit mal and idiopathic

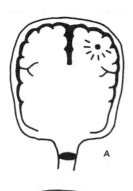

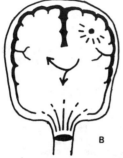

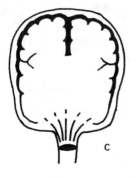

FIGURE 3 Classification of seizure disorders. A. _Focal seizure_ begins from a focal, unilateral part of the cortex (e.g., right-sided tonic movements, eyes deviated to one side, or an automatism of temporal lobe epilepsy). Most seizure disorders are focal, and almost all patients whose seizures begin after the age of 20 have a focal seizure disorder. B. _Focal seizure with secondary generalization_. Focal seizures may activate deep midline structures or spread to the other side, resulting in a bilateral generalized convulsion. The seizure disorder is still classified as a focal one, even though the focal element may have been transitory before the generalization. (EEG usually shows the focality.) C. _Primary generalized seizure_. No focal component is present either clinically or on EEG. These seizures represent true "idiopathic epilepsy" and usually begin before the age of 20 (e.g., petit mal, grand mal).

grand mal of children. A grand mal seizure is a major
motor seizure involving all extremities and having both
tonic and clonic features. It may represent a focal
seizure that has spread centrally and generalizes to
involve both hemisphere or it may begin as a generalized
seizure from the onset.

Major motor seizures may occur in normal individuals
secondary to drug withdrawal or metabolic factors (e.g.,
uremia, hypoglycemia). These may be focal or nonfocal
seizures, and are not felt to represent a true convulsive
disorder (see Chapters 22, 23).

ESTABLISH THE "FOCALITY"
OR "GENERALITY" OF THE DISORDER

History

1. Exactly how did the seizure start? Find a witness.
    Did the head and eyes turn? Were there other focal
    features?

2. At what age did the seizure begin? This is very
    important. Primary generalized seizures rarely begin
    before age 3 or after age 18. "Petit mal" that
    begins during adulthood is usually a temporal lobe
    absence attack.

3. Is there a family history of seizures? This may be
    present in both types but is more characteristic of
    generalized seizure disorders.

4. Was there focal trauma at birth or during an accident
    (head trauma)? Is there a history of a previous
    neurologic insult (e.g., stroke)?

5. Does the patient have abdominal pains, nausea,
    dizziness, behavioral disturbances, or automatisms
    (frequent features of temporal lobe epilepsy)? Are
    there déjà vu phenomena?

6. Is there a history of recent drug or alcohol
    ingestion or withdrawal?

7. Have there been brief staring spells not followed by
    postictal confusion or fatigue (petit mal epilepsy)?

EXAMINATION

A Search for Focal or Generalized Features

1. Look for postictal paralysis (Todd's paralysis) by
    checking for asymmetry of reflexes, hemiparesis,
    upgoing toes, or hemiparetic posturing of a foot
    (everted).

2. Are the eyes tonically deviated during the seizure?
    For example, a left hemisphere seizure drives the
    eyes to the right.

3. Look for asymmetry of fingernail, toe, and limb size
    (a clue to early damage of the contralateral
    hemisphere).

4. Arteriovenous malformations may present as focal
    seizures; listen for a bruit in any patient with
    unexplained seizures.

5. Petit mal (a primary generalized seizure disorder of
    childhood) can be precipitated by hyperventilation.
    Have the patient take up to 120 deep breaths and
    watch for a brief, transient cessation of activity
    and "glassy stare".

6. Examine the skin carefully. Neurocutaneous
    disorders, such as neurofibromatosis, tuberous
    sclerosis, and Sturge-Weber disease, may present with
    seizures.

LABORATORY AIDS IN DIAGNOSIS

1. In addition to baseline laboratory studies (including
    glucose, BUN, calcium, sodium), perform an EEG, brain
    scan or CAT scan, and LP for any unexplained first
    seizure. If the seizure was focal or a mass lesion
    is suspected, be sure there is no papilledema or
    midline shift before doing the LP.

2. Obtain a sleep EEG if a temporal lobe seizure
    disorder is suspected. Frequently, it will bring out
    the spike focus. In some cases the spike focus can
    only be seen with special (e.g., nasopharyngeal) EEG
    leads.

3. The decision to carry out further studies (e.g.,

arteriography) in a patient with focal seizures must
be made on an individual basis.

TREATMENT TIPS

Drugs for Focal Seizure Disorders

Phenytoin, phenobarbital, primidone (Mysoline), and
carbamazepine (Tegretol) are used to treat both adults and
children.   In adults, phenytoin is usually the first drug
administered.   In children, most begin with phenobarbital,
then add phenytoin, if necessary.   As a rule, do not use
two drugs unless one drug in adequate dosage (check blood
levels) has failed to control the seizures.

Drugs for Primary Generalized Seizure Disorders

Ethosuximide (Zarontin), valproic acid (Depakene),
phenytoin,   phenobarbital, acetazolamide (Diamox), and
clonezapam (Clonopin) are used.   Ethosuximide or valproic
acid are the drugs of choice for petit mal.   Although
primarily for the pediatric patient, ethosuximide and
acetazolamide can be beneficial in the adult who has had
primary generalized epilepsy since childhood or in those
with focal seizures and secondary spread.

Status Epilepticus

1. Maintain airway, administer O_2, prevent aspiration.

2. Draw blood to check metabolic parameters, especially
    glucose.   Start IV and administer 100 mg of thiamine
    followed by 50% glucose.

3. Diazepam (Valium) (10 mg slowly IV) is an effective
    first drug to stop seizures.   It can be repeated
    twice at 20-30 minute intervals.   Diazepam may cause
    respiratory arrest, especially in patients who have
    been given barbiturates and so should be used
    cautiously.   Diazepam may stop seizures, but it does
    not prevent further seizure activity or stop status
    epilepticus from beginning again.   Thus, after
    diazepam, administer diphenylhydantoin IV or
    phenobarbital IM for continued anticonvulsant
    control.

4. Phenytoin is an excellent drug for status

epilepticus (15 mg/kg IV over 30 to 45 minutes) and some physicians administer it as a first line drug (see below). It works well, does not depress respirations, and the patient is protected from further seizures. Hypotension can occur if the phenytoin is given too quickly. Thus, do not give faster than 50 mg per minute, and have blood pressure and EKG monitored periodically during IV administration. Use cautiously in patients with heart disease, especially those with conduction defects. For administration, phenytoin is best given undiluted or IV in saline; if given

// IV Dilantin must be
administered in saline //

in dextrose and water, it will precipitate.

5.   Sometimes, if diazepam and phenytoin are ineffective in status epilepticus, phenobarbital or paraldehyde may be necessary. If phenobarbital is given after phenytoin, it should be administered cautiously at a dose of 120 mg IM or IV, followed by 120 mg every 30 minutes until 300-500 mg have been given. Respiration and blood pressure must be watched carefully, particularly if the patient has received diazepam.

6.   Some physicians recommend giving phenytoin followed by phenobarbital for status epilepticus. If this is done, it is then very risky to administer diazepam because of possible respiratory arrest.

7.   If the combination of phenytoin and phenobarbital fails to stop status epilepticus, paraldehyde (10 cc per rectum, repeated q hour) may be tried, and if this fails, general anesthesia may be considered.

6.   When it proves difficult to control status epilepticus, there is often an underlying metabolic disorder (e.g., hyponatremia, hypoglycemia) or structural lesion (e.g., subdural, meningitis).

Phenytoin

1.   The average adult dose is 300-400 mg/day. Phenytoin can be given in one daily dose in adults, with the

patient maintaining blood levels in therapeutic range.

2. Therapeutic blood levels are 10 to 20 µg/ml; levels should be monitored in any patient who has not achieved good seizure control on phenytoin or other anticonvulsants.

3. Administered orally it takes 4 or 5 days to work; IV administration in adequate doses gives therapeutic levels within an hour. Patients may also be given loading doses orally, e.g., 500 mg b.i.d followed by daily maintenance doses. IM phenytoin is not absorbed evenly, causes muscle necrosis, and should be avoided.

4. Nystagmus on lateral gaze is a good clinical sign that the patient is taking his medication. Ataxia of gait and lethargy are common manifestations of toxicity.

5. Phenytoin is metabolized by the liver, so one can usually give regular doses to patients who have renal disease or are in renal failure.

6. A morbilliform rash occurs in about 4% of patients. If it is essential to use the drug, it is best to reduce the dose to a minimum and try to overcome the allergic reaction with the addition of antihistamines.

7. Other side effects include hirsutism, gum hypertrophy, megaloblastic anemia, osteomalacia, and lymphadenopathy. A teratogenic effect of phenytoin has been reported.

8. Warfarin and isoniazid (INH) enhance the action of phenytoin. Chronic administration of barbiturates may decrease blood phenytoin levels. Patients on phenytoin may have factitiously low thyroid function tests.

Phenobarbital

1. The average adult dose is 60 mg b.i.d.

2. Therapeutic blood levels are 20 to 40 µg/ml.

3.   Adults may not tolerate phenobarbital well because of its sedative effect, and children may develop behavioral abnormalities.

Primidone (Mysoline)

1.   Dosage: 125 to 250 mg, 3 to 4 times/day (10-25 mg/kg).

2.   Therapeutic blood levels are 5-12 μg/ml.

3.   Primidone must be introduced by small increments to avoid toxicity (oversedation, behavioral disturbances, and gastrointestinal [GI] dysfunction).

4.   A portion of primidone is metabolized to phenobarbital; thus, a combination of barbiturates and primidone often leads to oversedation.   Diazepam plus primidone may also cause oversedation.

Carbamazepine (Tegretol)

1.   Dosage: 200 mg, 3 to 4 times/day (7-15 mg/kg).

2.   Therapeutic blood levels are 4 to 8 μg/ml.

3.   Toxic side effects include leukopenia, hepatic dysfunction, and rashes. A period of reversible leukopenia usually precedes rare agranulocytosis.

4.   Carbamazepine is effective for psychomotor seizures and major motor seizures.

Valproic Acid (Depakene)

1.   Dosage: 250 mg, 3 to 4 times/day (15 mg/kg).

2.   Therapeutic blood levels are 50 to 100 μg/ml, although blood levels may correlate poorly with clinical response.

3.   Toxic effects include GI disturbances and sedation (especially if the dose is built up rapidly), ataxia, and liver dysfunction.

4.   Valproic acid is most effective in petit mal, myoclonic-akinetic seizures and primary generalized

epilepsies. It is structurally different than any
other anti-epileptic drug (a short chain branched
fatty acid).

5.   Interactions with other anticonvulsants include
     increased phenobarbital levels, and increased or
     decreased phenytoin levels.

        WHAT ETIOLOGIC FACTORS ARE INVOLVED?

     Metabolic factors, such as hypoglycemia,
hypocalcemia, or electrolyte imbalance may play a role at
any age. Other "metabolic causes" include uremia, hepatic
failure, and hypoxia.

     Drug withdrawal is a common cause of seizures in
adults (alcohol, barbiturates, and other sedatives).
Alcohol withdrawal seizures (rum fits) occur 12 to 48
hours after the cessation of drinking (see Chapter 22).
Alcoholics with post-traumatic epilepsy secondary to
frequent falls may have an exacerbation of seizures when
intoxicated.

     Exacerbation of a known seizure disorder is common.
A person with a controlled seizure disorder who comes to
the hospital because of a recurrence usually a) has not
been taking his medication (draw blood level); b) has been
drinking; or c) has an intercurrent infection. Change in
life style, emotional stress, or sleep deprivation may
also exacerbate seizures. Temporarily increase the
medication if seizures occur during a period of
intercurrent infection. Re-evaluate anyone with a
well-controlled seizure disorder that worsens with no
apparent cause.

     More than half of the cases of post-traumatic
epilepsy will develop during the first year after injury,
more than 80% by four years.

     Subdural hematoma can be associated with seizures
and must be considered in an alcoholic with new onset of
seizures.

     Etiology as related to age of onset:

     . Infancy and childhood: birth injury, congenital
       malformations, infectious, trauma, idiopathic

- Adolescence: idiopathic, trauma, drug-related

- Young adult: trauma, alcohol, neoplasm, drug-related

- Middle age: neoplasm, alcohol, vascular disease, trauma

- Late life (over 65):   vascular disease, neoplasm, degenerative

Note: Idiopathic or primary generalized epilepsy is generally apparent by age 18.   Seizures beginning after age 18 are usually due to a focal process or metabolic derangement.   Neoplasm is of prime concern during all of adult life.   After age 65, vascular disease (stroke) is the most common cause of a first seizure.

Remember

1) Check CBC periodically in patients on carbamazepine or ethosuximide and liver function in patients on Valproic acid.

2) Remind seizure patients of driving restrictions (which vary from state to state).

3) Don't stop anticonvulsants abruptly.

4) Alert patients to side effects of drugs.

REFERENCES

1.   Aminoff MJ, Simon RP: Status epilepticus: Causes, clinical features, and consequences in 98 patients. Am J Med 69:657, 1980.
2.   Annegers JF, Grabow JD, Graven RV, et al.:   Seizure after head trauma: Population study.   Neurology 30:683, 1980.
3.   Bear DM, Fedio P: Quantitative analysis of interictal behavior in temporal lobe epilepsy.   Arch Neurol 34:454, 1977.
4.   Delgado-Escueta AV, et al.:   Management of status epilepticus.   N Engl J Med 306:1337, 1982.
5.   Dichter MA: The epilepsies and convulsive disorders. In Harrison's Principles of Internal Medicine, New York, McGraw-Hill, 1983.

6. Goldensohn ES: Changing approaches to the management of seizures: pharmacologic considerations. *Epilepsia* 23, supplement 1, 1982.
7. Lennox WG, Lennox WA: *Epilepsy and Related Disorders*. Boston, Little, Brown and Company, 1960.
8. Schmidt R, Wilder B: *Epilepsy*. Philadelphia, F.A. Davis Company, 1968.
9. Solomon GE, Plum F: *Clinical Management of Seizures*. Philadelphia, W.B. Saunders, 1976.
10. Troupin A, Ojemann LM, Halpern L, et al.: Carbamazepine − A double blind comparison with phenytoin. *Neurology* 27:511, 1977.
11. Wilder BJ, Ramsay RE, Willmore LJ. et al.: Efficacy of intravenous phenytoin in the treatment of status epilepticus: Kinetics of central nervous system penetration. *Ann Neurol* 1:511, 1977.

Chapter 12

Vertigo-Dizziness

<u>Vertigo</u> implies the illusory sensation of turning or spinning; either of the patient himself or of his environment. <u>Dizziness</u> is less easily defined: light-headedness, giddiness, or a feeling of uneasiness in the head. Although vertigo may be distinguished from dizziness by demanding that unmistakable whirling or turning be present, these two symptoms are often not clinically distinguishable and may be approached as one entity. The goal of the clinician is to decide whether

// Is the process peripheral
central, or systemic //

the cause is <u>peripheral</u> (labyrinth, vestibular, or cochlear nerve), <u>central</u> (brainstem, cerebellum, or cerebral cortex), or <u>systemic</u> (e.g., cardiovascular, metabolic).

A careful history is often helpful in making this distinction.

HISTORY

1. Are the symptoms paroxysmal and are they related to head position?

2. Is there associated nausea, vomiting, headache?

3. Are symptoms of diplopia, dysarthria, numbness present?

4. Is there tinnitus? Deafness?

5.   Is there a lapse of awareness?

EXAMINATION OF THE PATIENT

1.   A general **physical** examination should include
     careful attention to the cardiovascular system (note
     arrhythmias).

2.   Specifically check the **ear canal** and **hearing**
     (listening to a watch tick, the spoken voice, and
     finger-rubbing screens three basic frequencies).

3.   Perform a complete **neurologic examination** with
     special attention to cranial nerves, cerebellar
     function, and the presence of nystagmus (horizontal
     or vertical).

4.   Check for **positional vertigo and nystagmus** by
     having the patient go from a sitting to supine
     position while quickly turning his head to the side.
     Note nystagmus, latency of the response, associated
     vertigo, and fatigability of the response.

5.   **Caloric testing** (minimal ice water caloric test).
     Patient lies supine with his head elevated 30
     degrees.   Irrigate each ear with 0.2 cc of ice water
     (use a tuberculin syringe).   Nystagmus (fast
     component) is in the direction of the opposite ear
     and should last about one minute.   (Formal calorics
     involve larger amounts of both warm and cold water.)
     The important point to notice is the symmetry or
     asymmetry between the response in each ear.

IS THE LESION PERIPHERAL OR CENTRAL?

   Peripheral lesions may be associated with deafness
and tinnitus (signs of eighth nerve dysfunction); there
are no central signs.   If the patient reports that caloric
testing reproduces his dizziness or he has a unilaterally
decreased caloric response, the lesion is peripheral.
Central lesions are defined by central nervous system
signs or symptoms (e.g., cerebellar ataxia, cranial nerve
abnormalities, diplopia, dysarthria, papilledema).
Vertigo of peripheral origin tends to parallel the
nystagmus   present.   In central lesions there is often
marked nystagmus with little or no vertigo; the
nystagmus is most prominent on looking toward the side

of the lesion and the fast component of the nystagmus
usually changes with looking in different directions. In
acute labyrinthine and vestibular nerve disorders, the
nystagmus is usually more prominent on looking toward the
good ear. In peripheral vestibulopathy, the patient falls
toward the side of the lesion and away from the fast
component of nystagmus. In central lesions, such as
cerebellar infarction, the patient falls toward the side
of the lesion and toward the fast component of
nystagmus.

Differentiation of Peripheral vs Central Nystagmus

	Peripheral	Central
Latency	3-10 sec.	None
Duration	60 sec.	60 sec.
Fatigability	Yes	No
Associated Symptoms	Nausea, vomiting	May have none
Vertical Nystagmus	Absent	May be present

Vertical nystagmus is a sign of brainstem disease
unless the patient is on medications (especially
barbiturates). Positional nystagmus of peripheral
origin usually begins three to ten seconds after assuming
the new head position (viz., latency of the response), is
commonly associated with vertigo and nausea, lasts up to
ten seconds, and is fatigable (it becomes harder to elicit
the nystagmus after several consecutive tries). Positional nystagmus of central origin begins immediately,
may last longer than ten seconds, and is not fatigable;
nausea and vertigo are not prominent. Rotary nystagmus
is generally seen with peripheral lesions.

IS THE LESION PERIPHERAL?

Middle ear disease may involve the labyrinth.
Check for otitis and other abnormalities of the tympanic
membrane. Establish whether the patient has been exposed

to ototoxic drugs. Remember, excessive wax in the ear can cause dizziness. Symptoms related to middle ear disease may be brought out by pressure applied to the external ear.

Menière's disease consists of a characteristic triad: vertigo, tinnitus, and deafness. The underlying mechanism probably relates to swelling of the endolymphatic space. Before vertigo appears there may be buildup with tinnitus and stuffiness; the attack itself is violent, with nausea and vomiting, sweating, and decreased hearing. Nystagmus is present only during the attack, and the direction may vary. Meniere's disease occurs in patients between the ages of 30 and 60, is a paroxysmal disorder, and is accompanied by residual tinnitus and hearing loss after multiple attacks. The vertigo lasts one to two hours, not seconds or days. Treatment includes sedatives, fluids, antihistamines, and antiemetics during the attack; prophylactically, some use diuretics and sodium restriction. Surgical therapy is recommended in some cases.

Benign paroxysmal positional vertigo, or episodic vertigo, occurs when the patient turns his head or changes position; it can be reproduced by testing for positional nystagmus (see above). There is no hearing loss, calorics are normal, and the disorder is self-limited. Treatment with meclizine is usually beneficial.

Acute labyrinthitis may be secondary to bacterial or viral infections. The onset may be sudden, with severe vertigo and gastrointestinal symptoms. The attack is not as short-lived as that of Meniere's disease, and lasts one to three days. There usually is spontaneous nystagmus toward the good ear, hearing may or may not be affected, and calorics are normal. Treatment is symptomatic, i.e., bed rest plus meclizine.

Vestibular neuronitis refers to sudden attacks of vertigo and nausea with no auditory signs or symptoms. Caloric testing shows hypofunction of the affected side, which serves to distinguish it from labyrinthitis. Treatment is symptomatic.

Post-traumatic vertigo is common and damage to the labyrinth is the postulated mechanism, since symptoms are those of peripheral vestibulopathy. The prognosis is good, with symptoms subsiding over a period of weeks.

DOES THE LESION BEGIN PERIPHERALLY
AND THEN SPREAD CENTRALLY?

Acoustic neuroma begins from sheath cells of the
vestibular portion of the eighth nerve in the internal
auditory canal; thus tinnitus, decreased hearing (e.g.,
trouble hearing on the phone), and dizziness or
disequilibrium are early complaints. As the tumor grows
into the cerebello-pontine angle, cranial nerve
dysfunction (loss of corneal reflex, facial weakness) and
cerebellar signs become prominent. Diagnosis is not
difficult once there is obvious CNS involvement. Early
recognition depends on ordering brainstem auditory evoked
responses and X-rays of the internal auditory canal in
patients with dizziness, unsteadiness, and/or symptoms
referrable to the eighth nerve (tinnitus and decreased
hearing). Sizable lesions of the acoustic nerve are
detectable by CAT scan. Small lesions are detectable by
posterior fossa myelography.

IS THE LESION CENTRAL?

Posterior fossa tumors may cause vertigo or
dizziness; look for cerebellar and other brainstem signs.
Check for evidence of raised intracranial pressure in
patients with "dizzy feelings" by examination of the
fundi.

// To establish vertebrobasilar
insufficiency, check for
brainstem symptoms or signs //

Vascular disease -- viz, vertebrobasilar
insufficiency -- may cause vertigo. To establish that
vertebrobasilar insufficiency is the cause, note other
brainstem symptoms (diplopia, slurred speech, numbness,
trouble swallowing), or signs (cranial nerve dysfunction,
motor or sensory loss). Other important points are:

1.   Dizziness or vertigo alone may be the first sign of
     vertebrobasilar insufficiency, but most patients have
     accompanying signs or symptoms of brainstem
     dysfunction within months of the onset of vertigo.

2.   The lateral medullary syndrome (see Chapter 6) may
     begin with vertigo.

3.   Cerebellar hemorrhage or infarction may begin with

the acute onset of dizziness, vomiting, inability to walk or stand, and severe headache (see Chapter 6).

4. Patients with the <u>subclavian steal syndrome</u> may experience attacks of vertigo (see Chapter 7).

5. If dizziness is accompanied by <u>eighth nerve dysfunction</u> only, it is probably not vascular in origin.

6. Vertigo is seldom a feature of carotid artery disease.

<u>Temporal lobe epilepsy</u> is an important cause of dizziness and vertigo. Note a history of staring spells, automatisms, déjà vu, or abdominal pain. Work-up for this seizure disorder should include a sleep EEG. Effective treatment is available (anticonvulsants).

Dizziness after <u>head trauma</u> may be nonspecific, benign paroxysmal vertigo, or represent post-traumatic epilepsy.

<u>Basilar migraine</u> may be associated with vertigo and is characterized by symptoms in the basilar artery territory. Check for vertigo, visual disturbances (including scotomata), tinnitus, blackouts, and associated complaints of throbbing occipital headache when the symptoms subside. Treatment includes prophylactic diphenylhydantoin, phenobarbital, or propranolol.

Check for a history of <u>diplopia</u>. Acute difficulty with eye movements may result in dizziness and/or vertigo. <u>Multiple sclerosis</u> may present with dizziness and/or diplopia due to brainstem involvement (see Chapter 15).

IS THE LESION SYSTEMIC?

Important causes to consider are cardiac arrhythmias, hyper- or hypotension, congestive heart failure, anemia, hypoglycemia, thyroid disease, and a variety of drugs (e.g., ototoxic drugs, anti-hypertensives, salicylates). Patients with multiple sensory deficits, e.g., poor vision and neuropathy, may complain of dizziness (this is seen most commonly in the elderly).

LABORATORY EVALUATION

Laboratory studies which may prove useful in the evaluation of the patient with vertigo/dizziness include: 1) auditory evoked responses, particularly sensitive for acoustic neuromas; and 2) electronystagmography, particularly sensitive for peripheral labyrinthopathies.

DIZZINESS AND/OR VERTIGO
WITH NO APPARENT CAUSE

Vertigo can be caused by psychogenic factors or be due to hyperventilation. In a study of a large series of patients who complained of dizziness, one of the most common causes was hyperventilation.

Occasionally, despite careful evaluation, a patient's dizziness appears to be idiopathic. In these circumstances, symptomatic treatment and careful follow-up of the patient is required.

TREATMENT

Drugs that may be useful in the treatment of dizziness/vertigo include: meclizine, diazepam, anti-histamines, and anticholinergics. The patient should also be advised to avoid sudden positional changes.

REFERENCES

1.   Bickerstaff ER: Basilar artery migraine. Lancet 1:15, 1961.
2.   Brandt T, Daroff RB: The multisensory physiological and pathological vertigo syndromes. Ann Neurol 7:195, 1980.
3.   Drachman D, Hart C: An approach to the dizzy patient. Neurology 22:323, 1972.
4.   Nelson JR: The minimal ice water caloric test. Neurology 19:577, 1969.
5.   Symposium on vertigo. Otolaryngol Clin N Amer 6(1), Feb, 1973.
6.   Troost BT: Dizziness and vertigo in vertibrobasilar disease. In Current Concepts of Cerebrovascular Disease 14:(5)(6), 1979.
7.   Wolfson R: Vertigo. CIBA Clinical Symposium, Vol 33(6), 1981.

Chapter 13

Sleep Disorders

Sleep disorders are more common than generally realized. Approximately 10-15% of the population have sleep related problems. Early diagnosis and proper treatment depends on alertness to characteristic signs and symptoms by the primary care physician. Most persistent sleep problems are characterized by excessive sleepiness and/or by difficulty initiating or maintaining sleep. Excessive sleepiness or drowsiness during the day may include falling asleep during activities such as eating, driving, or while sitting in a class.

In addition to sleepiness, patients with <u>narcolepsy</u> have one or more of the following:

1. <u>Cataplexy</u> - sudden loss of muscle tone, induced by emotion or sudden stimuli.

2. <u>Sleep attacks</u> - uncontrollable attacks of sleep for short periods.

3. <u>Sleep paralysis</u> - upon waking or in transition to sleep, the patient is unable to move.

4. <u>Hypnogogic or hypnopompic hallucinations</u> - false visual or auditory perceptions just before falling asleep, or when just awakening.

Patients with the **sleep apnea** syndrome may have the following:

. Restless sleep, enuresis, impotence, morning headaches, memory disturbances, learning problems, heavy snoring, and hypertension.

In **insomnia**, the patient cannot fall asleep at night, has difficulty staying asleep and/or wakes up early. Disturbed nocturnal sleep leads to daytime drowsiness.

Important points to explore in the **history** include:

a. Does the patient wake up feeling refreshed, even after a short nap? (narcolepsy)

b. Observations by the patient's sleep partner. Is the patient's sleep restless? Are there pauses of more than ten seconds between breaths? Is there choking, gagging, or snorting (sleep apnea)?

c. Are there symptoms of **depression**, including poor appetite, early awakening, weight loss, sadness, suggesting a secondary sleep disorder?

d. Does the patient have chronic renal failure or chronic alcoholism, each of which has been associated with secondary sleep disorders?

e. Are there symptoms of anxiety which are disturbing sleep, or are there other psychiatric abnormalities ("psychiatric insomnia")?

Examination of patients with sleep disorders is usually normal. However, special attention should be paid to:

a. Body habitus and neck size -- middle-aged patients with sleep apnea frequently are obese men with thick necks. Sometimes enlarged tonsils or other pharyngeal abnormalities can contribute to obstructive sleep apnea.

b. Memory -- frequently impaired in patients with sleep apnea.

c.   Retro- or micrognathia (jaw abnormalities)
      predispose to sleep apnea.

d.   Stigmata of hypothyroidism or acromegaly.

f.   Hypertension and arrhythmias (especially
      nocturnal) -- seen in sleep apnea.

Laboratory studies of patients with sleep disorders
depend on the suspected diagnosis:

In narcolepsy a sleep electroencephalogram (EEG)
combined with electromyographic (EMG) and electro-
oculographic (EOG) monitoring is frequently abnormal,
showing rapid eye movements (REM) sleep at sleep outset
rather than later in the sleep cycle.

In suspected sleep apnea a record of the patient's
breathing pattern during sleep is necessary. Monitoring
of O_2, CO_2 exchange by mask, and diaphragmatic motion can
help distinguish obstructive from central from mixed
types of sleep apnea.

TREATMENT

1.   Weight loss, treatment with respiratory stimulants,
      tonsillectomy, and, if necessary, tracheostomy may be
      indicated in the treatment of obstructive sleep
      apnea. Diaphragmatic pacing is used in the central
      type.

2.   Frequent naps and use of stimulant drugs, such as
      pemoline and methylphenidate, are used in narcolepsy.
      Tricyclic antidepressants, such as clomipramine,
      are useful in cataplexy.

3.   The treatment of insomnias is difficult and must be
      tailored to the individual patient. Modalities
      include:

      .   Environmental manipulation (e.g., altering bedtime
           routine, evening exercise, hot baths before sleep)

      .   Relaxation techniques

      .   Psychotherapy

      .   Short-term hypnotic drug use

Other less common sleep disorders include somnambulism (sleep walking), night terrors and nightmares, enuresis, nocturnal myoclonus.

REFERENCES

1.   Kales A, Kales JD: Sleep disorders. Recent findings in the diagnosis and treatment of disturbed sleep. N Engl J Med 290:487, 1974.
2.   Guilleminault C, Dement WC: 235 cases of excessive daytime sleepiness. J Neurol Sci 31:13, 1977.
3.   Pagel JF: Sleep disorders and insomnia. Am Fam Physician 17:165, 1978.

Chapter 14

Spinal Cord Compression

Acute spinal cord compression is a neurologic emergency. Prognosis is clearly related to the delay between onset of neurologic symptoms and treatment.

CHARACTERISTIC SYMPTOMS

- Back pain

- Paresthesias in legs ("funny feelings", tingling, or numbness)

- Change in urine function (patient urinates more or less frequently)

- Weakness in lower extremities (especially in climbing stairs)

- Constipation

EARLY SIGNS

- Loss of pinprick sensation or a different reaction to pinprick in the lower extremities. The patient may or may not have a sensory "level" to pinprick. There may be a temperature "level" to a cool object.

- Position or vibration loss in the feet

- Slight hyperreflexia in the lower extremities as compared to the upper (Note: the toes are often downgoing and reflexes reduced in early acute cord compression).

- Tenderness over the spine is a helpful sign in determining the level of the lesion.

LATE SIGNS

- Definite weakness

- Definite hyperreflexia

- Upgoing toes

- A sensory level to pinprick, temperature and/or vibration. It is often helpful to check vibration sense up and down the spine in search of a level.

- Loss of anal sphincter tone, absent abdominal reflexes

- Urinary retention

CAUSES OF SPINAL CORD COMPRESSION

Epidural Compression

- Metastatic tumor (especially from lung and breast)

- Trauma

- Lymphoma

- Multiple myeloma

- Epidural abscess or hematoma

- Cervical or thoracic disk protrusion or spondylosis

- Atlanto-axial subluxation (rheumatoid arthritis)

Extra-arachnoid, Intradural Compression

- Meningioma

- Neurofibroma

Intramedullary Expansion

- Glioma

. Ependymoma

. Arteriovenous malformation

DIAGNOSTIC STEPS

1. Perform a careful neurologic examination; estimate the level of the cord lesion.

2. Check for primary tumor sites (e.g., careful breast examination, prostate examination, chest X-ray, routine laboratory studies, including CBC, uric acid).

3. Plain films of the spine should be obtained and may reveal (a) vertebral collapse or subluxation, (b) bony erosion secondary to tumor, or (c) calcification (meningioma).

4. Early consultation with a neurologist and/or neuro-surgeon is needed.

5. Do not perform an LP if cord compression is suspected; CSF will be examined in conjunction with myelography.

TREATMENT

Treatment depends on the site(s) of cord block and the etiology. Modalities include radiotherapy (for such disorders as Hodgkin's lymphoma), surgical decompression for solitary radioresistant extradural solid tumors, or a combination of both.

Dexamethasone (10 mg-50 mg IV) is usually given immediately (before myelography, radiotherapy, or surgery) when compression is suspected clinically, as it may help preserve spinal cord function.

NOTE:

1. Transverse myelitis is characterized by the acute or subacute development of paraplegia, occasionally asymmetrical, associated with back pain and sensory loss. It may or may not be related to a preceding viral illness (e.g., mononucleosis). The CSF may show pleocytosis with increased protein and normal sugar. Myelography is usually necessary to rule out a

compressive lesion. Treatment is supportive.
Corticosteroids are often used when the etiology is
thought to be post-infectious and/or demyelinating.

2. Radiation myelopathy usually occurs six months to a
    year following irradiation to the thoracic area of
    the spinal cord (e.g., for lymphoma). Onset may be
    insidious or abrupt and may be limited to
    paresthesias or progress to actual paralysis. There
    is no known treatment and the myelopathy is probably
    secondary to vascular damage to the spinal cord.
    Myelography is needed to rule out a compressive
    lesion. (Occasionally, radiation myelopathy may
    occur years following therapy.)

3. Myelopathy may also be secondary to toxins (e.g.,
    heroin, arsenic), associated with malignancy
    elsewhere in the body as a remote effect, or
    secondary to vascular infarction of the spinal cord
    (see p. 37).

REFERENCES

1. Baker AS, Ojemann RG, Swartz MN, Richardson EP:
    Spinal epidural abscess. N Engl J Med 293:463,
    1975.
2. Gilbert R, Posner JB: Extradural spinal cord
    compression from metastatic cancer: diagnosis and
    treatment. Neurology 27:366, 1977.
3. Rodriguez M, Dinapoli R: Epidural cord compression
    with special reference to metastatic epidural tumors.
    Mayo Clin Proc 55:442, 1980.
4. Ropper WD, Poskanzer DC: The prognosis of acute and
    sub-acute transverse myelopathy based on early signs
    and symptoms. Ann Neurol 4:51, 1978.
5. Tobin WD, Layton DD: The diagnosis and natural
    history of spinal cord arteriovenous malformations.
    Mayo Clin Proc 51:637, 1976.

Chapter 15

Hyperreflexia and Hyporeflexia

Normal reflexes suggest that the motor system between cortex and muscle is functioning normally. Pathologically hyperactive reflexes imply disease between cortex and spinal cord, and hypoactive reflexes imply disease between spinal cord and muscle.

HYPERREFLEXIA

Hyperreflexia signifies an upper motor neuron lesion along the neuraxis from cortex to lateral columns of the spinal cord. When anterior horn cell or peripheral nerve are involved, there is usually hyporeflexia.

// Hyperactive reflexes in
the presence of downgoing
toes are usually normal //

Many people have exaggerated reflexes that may appear hyperactive. A good rule is that symmetrical hyperactive reflexes in the presence of downgoing toes are usually normal. If the hyperactive reflexes truly reflect pyramidal tract disease, the toes should also be abnormal. Abdominal reflexes (stroke skin next to umbilicus) may be absent on the side of pyramidal tract dysfunction. Check for a brisk jaw jerk in patients with hyperreflexia; its presence suggests bilateral lesions above the midpons.

A unilaterally upgoing toe, or <u>hyperactive reflexes</u>
<u>on one side</u> implies damage to one side of the nervous
system. Decide whether this represents an old lesion
not requiring further investigation or a newly developing
one. Check for:

1. <u>History of birth injury</u>. An otherwise normal
    person may have unilateral hyperreflexia with no
    apparent cause. This may be due to birth injury with
    mild cerebral palsy.

2. <u>Old neurologic disease</u>. A patient with a history
    of meningitis, stroke, subdural hematoma, etc., may
    have unilateral hyperreflexia. Remember, a small
    stroke may not have been recognized by the patient.

3. <u>Newly developing signs or symptoms</u>. If history
    suggests this, a full investigation is warranted.

Bilateral Hyperreflexia

Bilateral hyperreflexia with upgoing toes implies
bilateral pyramidal tract dysfunction. Note the
following:

1. With <u>spinal cord compression</u> look for metastatic
    disease in the adult, intrinsic tumor in the younger
    person, or bony abnormalities of the spine, all of
    which may cause bilateral hyperreflexia. Carefully
    check for sensory level, local back tenderness, and
    other features of spinal cord compression (Chapter
    14).

2. <u>Cervical spondylosis</u> is the most common cause of
    spinal cord dysfunction in older people. Ask about
    neck pain. Look for bilateral hyperreflexia, muscle
    wasting in arms and/or hands, decreased range of
    motion of the neck, and degenerative changes on X-ray
    of the cervical spine (see Chapter 18).

3. <u>Multiple sclerosis</u> (MS) is an important cause of
    hyperreflexia in a young person. The reflexes may be
    markedly increased and in some instances there may be
    unilateral hyperreflexia. These patients may not
    have noticed the transitory episode that caused the
    hyperreflexia; however, a careful history and
    examination usually delineates a story suggestive of
    multiple sclerosis:

- MS may take one of two forms: 1) **relapsing, remitting** disease of the nervous system, there are "multiple lesions in time and space"; 2) **chronic progressive disease**, usually progressive spinal cord dysfunction.

- Common **symptoms**: unilateral loss of vision that has resolved (optic neuritis), bladder disturbances (incontinence), sensory symptoms (heaviness or numbness in an extremity), diplopia, speech and gait difficulties.

- Frequent **physical findings**: pallor of the optic disc, internuclear ophthalmoplegia, cerebellar ataxia, dysarthria, hyperreflexia, spasticity and weakness of lower extremities.

- **Diagnosis** is based on history and physical examination and spinal fluid abnormalities that include elevated gamma globulin and the presence of oligoclonal banding. A very helpful laboratory study is measurement of visual, auditory, and somatosensory evoked responses (at least 75% of MS patients have abnormal visual evoked responses [VER], even those patients without visual symptoms). Abnormal VER's may establish the diagnosis in a patient with only spinal cord abnormalities by identifying a "second lesion" in the nervous system. Abnormalities of suppressor T lymphocytes appear to parallel disease activity.

- Treatment is primarily supportive; steroids are usually given during acute exacerbations. The use of short-term intensive immunosuppression with high-dose cyclophosphamide may be of benefit in stabilizing patients with actively progressive disease (NEJM 308:173, 1983).

Remember that spinal cord compression is an important differential diagnosis in the patient with possible multiple sclerosis, and a myelogram is often performed to rule out surgically correctable lesions.

4. **Multiple small strokes** (état lacunaire) can cause bilateral hyperreflexia and is frequently seen in the elderly patient with hypertension or diabetes. Check for a history of multiple, small CVAs (although they

may have been clinically silent) as well as other evidence of vascular disease. Search for other associated signs of "multiple stroke" syndrome: emotional lability, increased jaw jerk, increased gag reflex (features of pseudobulbar palsy), and ataxia. In addition, there may be dementia with memory impairment (see Chapter 10).

5.   Familial spastic paraplegia is a cause of hyperreflexia; be sure to check the family history.

6.   Metabolic causes of hyperreflexia include hepatic and uremic encephalopathy.

7.   Amyotrophic lateral sclerosis (ALS) causes increased reflexes secondary to pyramidal tract involvement. This may occur in brainstem (increased jaw jerk) and/or spinal cord. In addition, fasciculations and muscle wasting occur due to associated anterior horn cell disease (e.g., fasciculations of the tongue). The combination of upper and lower motor neuron signs in spinal cord and brainstem without sensory loss is virtually diagnostic of ALS.

8.   Hyperreflexia can be seen in otherwise normal anxious patients.

NOTE: Hyperreflexia in both arms and legs implies a lesion at the cervical cord or higher; hyperreflexia in the legs only implies a lesion below the cervical cord. There are three exceptions to this basic anatomic rule:

1. Cerebral palsy. Leg fibers may be selectively involved in the white matter of the hemispheres, giving increased reflexes in legs only ("spastic diparesis").

2. Parasagittal intracranial mass. By virtue of its location, it may affect cortical leg fibers, producing hyperreflexia in legs only, mimicking a cord lesion. Headache, seizures, and/or papilledema may be present.

3. Hydrocephalus may present with spastic paraparesis because parasagittal leg fibers are stretched most by dilated lateral ventricles. Arnold-Chiari malformation may be associated with a spastic paraparesis.

HYPOREFLEXIA

Hyporeflexia usually indicates peripheral nerve disease with one component of the reflex pathway being abnormal: peripheral nerve, sensory root, anterior horn cells in cord, motor root, or muscle. Reflexes can be reinforced by having the patient pull his hands apart or bite down when reflexes are tested. Areflexia implies no reflexes, even with reinforcement; reflexes present only with reinforcement imply an intact reflex pathway and may or may not be abnormal. Consider the following points when confronted with hyporeflexia:

Normally hypoactive reflexes. Occasionally one sees otherwise normal individuals with hyporeflexia and no obvious cause.

Delayed relaxation phase of the reflex. This unique "hypoactive" reflex is classic for hypothyroidism and at times serves as the first clue to this metabolic abnormality (it is best seen in the ankle jerk).

Spinal shock. This is a very important cause of areflexia and is often seen during the initial stages of cord damage -- whether traumatic, vascular, or neoplastic in origin. Although compressive damage to spinal cord generally causes hyperactive reflexes, remember that acutely (during the first days, and often as long as one to two weeks), reflexes may be depressed or absent. Be sure to check for a sensory level, especially if there is leg weakness.

Acute stroke. Initially, there is usually hyporeflexia on the side of the hemiparesis; later, hyperreflexia develops.

Asymptomatic areflexia with a large pupil. This is a benign syndrome (Adie's), consisting of generalized areflexia plus a large pupil that reacts to accommodation but not to direct light.

Myopathy. Muscle disorders may cause hyporeflexia (although usually not areflexia). Remember, weakness from muscle disease is generally proximal (shoulder and hip), while weakness from peripheral nerve disease is more marked distally (hand and foot).

Isolated unilaterally absent reflex. This is a
very important sign of disc disease compressing spinal
roots and can be seen with diseases affecting specific
peripheral nerves. Some examples:

1. _Unilaterally absent ankle jerk_ should arouse
    suspicion of disc disease with compression of the S1
    root on the same side. (Ask the patient about
    sciatic pain and check straight leg raising.)
    Similarly, but less frequently, the knee jerk may be
    absent unilaterally with root disease at L3 or L4 or
    with femoral neuropathy (see Chapter 19).

2. _Unilaterally absent brachioradialis, biceps or_
    triceps reflex may imply impingement on C5, C6, or
    C7 nerve roots in the cervical region from cervical
    spondylosis.

3. Remember, _mononeuropathy or plexus injury_, whether
    traumatic or from tumor, are other important causes
    of asymmetrical reflex loss (see Chapter 19).

> // If the patient has no
> reflexes, he usually has
> a neuropathy //

Bilateral areflexia is the hallmark of
neuropathies, a broad category of diseases affecting
peripheral nerves. If one cannot elicit reflexes in a
patient, he usually has a neuropathy. Neuropathies may be
categorized into motor and sensory neuropathies, although
there is considerable overlap, and often a "sensorimotor"
neuropathy.

1. _Areflexia with acute or subacutely developing motor_
    weakness and little sensory loss is the classic
    presentation of the _Guillain-Barré syndrome_, or
    acute inflammatory polyneuritis. The patient has
    tingling or "funny feelings" in his hands and feet,
    although motor weakness exceeds the sensory symptoms.
    Inflammatory polyneuritis may begin days to weeks
    after a systemic infection (usually viral),
    immunization, or can follow such nonspecific factors
    as a surgical procedure.

    a. _Clinical characteristics_. In the _mild_ form
        the patient's motor difficulties are confined to
        problems with gait and trouble using the

upper extremities. The dysfunction does not progress, and a clue to the diagnosis is the areflexia. The **moderate** form is an extension of the mild form but includes enough weakness that the patient is now unable to walk alone. In the **severe** form, the ascending weakness becomes an ascending paralysis that includes respiratory muscles, and involvement of cranial nerves. These patients require tracheostomy and intensive respiratory care. **Autonomic dysfunction** may occur causing fluctuations in blood pressure, temperature, and heart rate. Some patients may die, but most recover and are able to walk again.

b. **Diagnosis.** Clinical features include an ascending progressive muscle weakness that is more prominent proximally, **areflexia**, a mild distal sensory loss, and bilateral facial weakness (an important clue). An LP usually shows: raised CSF protein without pleocytosis. CSF protein may be normal during the initial stage of the illness but usually rises later. Nerve conduction velocities are abnormal early in the course of the disease.

c. **Treatment.** In Guillain-Barré syndrome, the severity of the paralysis may not be evident at first. Therefore the physician must recognize that he is dealing with acute inflammatory polyneuritis and carefully monitor respiratory function, including blood gases and vital capacity, until the paralysis has reached a plateau. This is crucial. The benefit of steroids is controversial, although a course of steroids is often initiated if the patient is deteriorating or not improving. A recent treatment modality whose efficacy remains to be established is plasmapheresis. The mainstay of treatment is supportive, including meticulous pulmonary and nursing care and treating of autonomic dysfunction, including arrhythmias.

d. **Differential diagnosis.** Check for porphyria, botulism, polyarteritis, toxin exposure, and diphtheria (palatal and extraocular muscle palsies); these processes may mimic the Guillain-Barré syndrome. Also, test for mononucleosis, hepatitis, and mycoplasma infection, one of which may have been preceding illness.

2. <u>Areflexia with sensory neuropathy and little or late developing motor loss</u>:

    a. <u>Diabetes</u>. Various neuropathies may be associated with diabetes (see Chapter 20); most common is a bilateral symmetrical neuropathy manifested by absent ankle jerks and decreased vibration sense. Motor weakness is minimal.

    b. <u>Alcoholism</u> (nutritional and toxic deficit). These patients have a sensory neuropathy involving feet and hands, including decreased vibration sense (see Chapter 23). They have numbness and tingling, and their feet are very tender to touch. Weakness is minimal, although this distal sensory neuropathy occasionally progresses to an incapacitating motor neuropathy.

    c. <u>Vitamin B$_{12}$ deficiency</u> may produce lower limb areflexia and distal paresthesias.

    d. <u>Uremia</u>. The patient often has "restless legs" and may develop profound distal sensory loss with muscle atrophy, areflexia, and burning sensations (see Chapter 22).

    e. <u>Tumors</u> (especially lung). Malignancy may have, as its initial manifestation, a relatively pure sensory neuropathy with numbness, paresthesias, and ataxia of hands and feet; motor involvement may appear later. Always check for occult malignancy in the patient with a sensory neuropathy of unknown etiology.

    f. <u>Amyloid</u>, almost invariably associated with a blood dyscrasia or tumor, can present with a sensory neuropathy with autonomic manifestations.

    g. <u>Note</u>: A familial sensory radicular neuropathy with autosomal dominant inheritance may present during the second and third decades. Fabry's and Refsum's disease may present as a sensory neuropathy.

3. <u>Bilateral areflexia and neuropathy on a familial basis</u>. The prototype for familial neuropathy is <u>Charcot-Marie-Tooth disease</u> (peroneal muscular

atrophy). These patients have sensory loss,
"champagne-bottle" legs, a wide-spread areflexia not
merely confined to the ankles, and pes cavus.
Familial neuropathies may be associated with other
inherited neurologic diseases, with other symptoms
being present: e.g., cerebellar tremor, nystagmus,
and ataxia.

Work-up of Neuropathies

In most instances the etiology of a patient's
neuropathy can be determined, particularly with intensive
evaluation. Check these important points when dealing
with a neuropathic process of undetermined cause:

1. Is there evidence of <u>toxin exposure</u>: arsenic
    (painful red feet, gastrointestinal disturbances),
    thallium (alopecia), lead (affects upper extremities,
    including motor neuropathies with wrist drop, and
    causes lead line in gums), other metals (copper,
    zinc, mercury)? Consider organic toxins and
    occupational exposures.

2. Check for <u>drugs</u> that may cause neuropathy.
    Nitrofurantoin, isoniazid, and vincristine are common
    offenders. Check each medication the patient takes.

3. Does the patient have an associated <u>systemic
    illness</u>: hypothyroidism, syphilis, amyloid (large
    tongue, gastrointestinal symptoms), myeloma or other
    gammopathy, leprosy (anesthetic skin patches), lupus,
    sarcoid, polyarteritis, pernicious anemia, or
    porphyria?

4. Is the neuropathy <u>relapsing</u>? An important group is
    the idiopathic type of polyneuritis which responds to
    steroids; other relapsing neuropathies may be due to
    alcohol ingestion, porphyria, or lead poisoning.

5. Have <u>nerve conduction studies</u> performed when the
    diagnosis is in doubt; nerve conduction velocities
    are decreased in peripheral neuropathy and may be
    normal or mildly reduced in axonal neuropathy.
    Depending on the neuropathy, motor and sensory
    conductions may be differentially affected.

6. <u>Nerve biopsy</u> is sometimes diagnostic (e.g.,
    amyloid).

Treatment of Neuropathies

Removal of the offending agent in toxic neuropathies and, where possible, treatment of an associated systemic illness are important. Vitamin replacement is indicated in deficiency states. Steroids are useful in relapsing polyneuritis and polyarteritis and may be useful in acute infectious polyneuritis.

Note: A mneumonic device that may aid in remembering causes of neuropathy is "DAG THERAPIST".

D = diabetes	T = toxins
A = alcohol	He = hereditary
G = Guillain-Barré	R = Refsum's
	A = amyloid
	P = porphyria
	I = infection
	S = systemic
	T = tumor

REFERENCES

1. Asbury AK, Aranson BG, Adams RD: The inflammatory lesion in idiopathic polyneuritis. _Medicine_ 48:173, 1969.
2. Dyck PJ, et al.: Intensive evaluation of referred unclassified neuropathies yields improved diagnosis. _Ann Neurol_ 10:222, 1981.
3. Dyck PJ, Lais AC, Ohta M, et al.: Chronic inflammatory polyradiculoneuropathy. _Mayo Clin Proc_ 50:621, 1975.
4. Dyck PJ, Lambert EH: Lower motor and primary sensory neuron disease with peroneal muscular atrophy. _Arch Neurol_ 18:603, 609, 1968.
5. Dyck PJ, Thomas PK, Lambert EH: _Peripheral Neuropathy_. Philadelphia, W.B. Saunders Company, 1975.
6. McFarlin DE, McFarland HF: Multiple sclerosis. _N Engl J Med_ 307:1183, 1246, 1982.
7. Swick HM, McQuillen MP: The use of steroids in the treatment of idiopathic polyneuritis. _Neurology_ 26:205, 1976.
8. Wilkinson M: _Cervical Spondylosis: Its Early Diagnosis and Treatment_. Philadelphia, W.B. Saunders Company, 1971.

Chapter 16

Myopathy

When confronted with a patient who may have a myopathy, the physician must establish whether the weakness is indeed myopathic, if the myopathy is congenital or acquired, and if acquired, whether it represents a manifestation of another illness (e.g., thyroid myopathy).

THE HISTORY

In a patient complaining of weakness in whom the diagnosis of myopathy is made, one finds:

1. The weakness is <u>gradual</u> rather than sudden in onset and is symmetrical.

2. There are no paresthesias or "pins and needles" feeling in the limbs.

3. Climbing stairs and combing hair are particularly difficult (<u>proximal weakness</u>).

4. Bowel and bladder function are not affected.

5. The weakness is usually painless.

Establish the following points:

1. Is there a <u>family history</u> of a similar disorder?

2. Is there myotonia (inability to release grip)?

3. Is there trouble swallowing (polymyositis) or variation in the weakness that occurs during the day (myasthenia).

103

TABLE 2   MYOPATHIC AND RELATED DISORDERS

Acquired myopathies

. Polymyositis (idiopathic or associated with tumor)

. Thyroid

. Steroid associated

. Alcoholic

Muscular dystropies (onset after age 30 is rare)

. Duchenne: affects young boys, death by age 20

. Fascioscapulohumeral: autosomal dominant, onset
between age 10 and 20

. Limb-girdle: affects shoulder and pelvis
musculature, onset between age 15 and 25

. Myotonic dystrophy: usually manifests in early
adult life with myotonia, peripheral muscle wasting,
impotence, frontal balding, cataracts; inheritance is
autosomal dominant

Myasthenia gravis: classically involves ocular muscles;
fatigability and variability are characteristic; there may
be proximal muscle weakness.

4. What was the exact age of onset? This may help to distinguish congenital from acquired myopathies.

PHYSICAL EXAMINATION

The myopathic patient presents these findings:

1. <u>Proximal limb strength</u> is more impaired than distal strength (except in myotonic dystrophy). Check deltoids (shoulder) and iliopsoas (hips). Weakness tends to be <u>distal</u> in neuropathies. Weakness may be proximal in Guillain-Barre but there are areflexia, sensory symptoms, and raised CSF protein.

2. <u>Neck flexion</u> is much weaker than neck extension.

3. <u>Reflexes</u> are preserved or slightly decreased except in late stages of disease.

4. <u>Sensation</u> is unimpaired. This is <u>not</u> true in neuropathies.

Check these points which help distinguish one myopathy from another.

1. Note whether <u>facial muscles</u> are involved. Have patient shut eyes tight, puff cheeks, or attempt to whistle (difficult in fascioscapulohumeral).

2. Check for <u>fatigability</u>, especially of extraocular movements. Practically all patients with myasthenia gravis have ptosis or diplopia at some time in the course of their illness.

3. See if <u>pelvic</u> and <u>thigh muscles</u> are more involved than those of the head and shoulders (limb-girdle).

4. Check for <u>myotonia</u> by percussing the thenar eminence or the tongue and check for lid myotonia by having the patient shut his eyes tightly and then quickly open them. Patients with myotonia may be unable to "let go" after handshake.

LABORATORY STUDIES

Characteristic features of myopathies include:

. Elevated muscle enzymes, especially CPK.   SGOT, aldolase, and LDH may also be elevated.

. Normal spinal fluid, including the protein level.

Special studies usually done on the patient suspected of myopathic disease include:

. Electromyogram (EMG)

. Muscle biopsy

IS THERE A TREATABLE MYOPATHY PRESENT?

Check for the following:

1.   Thyroid myopathy (both hyper- and hypothyroidism).

2.   Steroid myopathy. Has the patient been on steroids for another disorder? (Fluorinated steroids are especially prone to cause steroid induced myopathy.) Does he have Cushing's disease?

3.   Idiopathic polymyositis. There is usually an elevated sedimentation rate and, at times, evidence of other connective tissue disease, such as dermatomyositis, rheumatoid arthritis, or lupus. Treatment is with steroids.

4.   Polymyositis associated with malignancy. Some adults with polymyositis will have the symptoms as a remote effect of cancer. Polymyositis may also be associated with sarcoid.

5.   Alcoholic myopathy. Check for a history of alcoholism. Does the patient have an associated cardiac myopathy?

6.   Periodic paralysis. Attacks are often related to cold, food, or exercise. Check the serum potassium level during an attack.

7.   **Polymyalgia rheumatica**. Although this disorder is
     not associated with muscle weakness, patients
     complain of muscle and joint aches. The
     sedimentation rate is elevated and the disorder is
     exquisitely responsive to steroids.

8.   **Myasthenia gravis**. Does the patient have
     fluctuating weakness during the day? The diagnosis
     of myasthenia is usually confirmed by a Tensilon test
     or repetitive nerve stimulation. Treatment involves
     use of anticholinesterases, prednisone, thymectomy,
     and in some cases plasmapheresis. Myasthenia,
     usually classified with myopathies, is actually a
     disease of the neuromuscular junction. The etiology
     relates to a post-synaptic defect of acetylcholine
     receptors at the neuromuscular junction, caused by
     circulating antibodies and thymus-derived lymphocytes
     directed against the acetylcholine receptor. The
     presence of anti-acetylcholine receptor antibodies in
     the blood is highly specific for myasthenia gravis.

REFERENCES

1.   Walton JN: **Disorders of Voluntary Muscle**. 3rd ed,
     London, Churchill Livingstone, 1974.
2.   Dubowitz V and Brooke MH: **Muscle Biopsy: A Modern
     Approach**. London, WB Saunders, 1973.
3.   Bohan A and Peter J: Polymyositis and
     dermatomyositis, **N Engl J Med** 292:344, 1975.
4.   Swift TR: Disorders of neuromuscular transmission
     other than myasthenia gravis. **Muscle and Nerve**
     4:334, 1981.
5.   Brooke MH: **A Clinician's View of Neuromuscular
     Diseases**, Baltimore, Williams & Wilkins, 1977.
6.   Drachman DB: Myasthenia gravis. **N Engl J Med**
     298:136, 186, 1978.

Chapter 17

Tremor

Tremor involves rhythmic oscillating movement of the extremities or head. Types of tremor include: (1) action tremor of the essential, familial, or senile type; (2) resting tremor associated with Parkinson's disease, (3) intention tremor associated with cerebellar dysfunction (e.g., brought out by "finger-to-nose" movement of an extremity). Other disorders of movement are also discussed in this chapter.

ACTION TREMOR

Action tremor is a tremor of posture or activity that disappears at rest; it is usually asymmetrical. Some people may be unable to sign their name in public or lift a cup to their lips because of exacerbation of the tremor with anxiety or use of the arms. Patients may have an associated head tremor, although seldom is there a head tremor without an arm tremor; legs are rarely involved. Action tremor is of lower amplitude than Parkinsonian tremor and is unaccompanied by the rigidity and the slowness (bradykinesia) of Parkinson's disease. Action tremor may be familial, senile or "essential", and may be helped temporarily by alcohol ingestion (a diagnostic maneuver). Neurologic examination is otherwise normal in patients with action tremor. <u>Differential Diagnosis</u>: Action tremor may be associated with pheochromocytoma, hyperthyroidism, toxins, and with administration of amphetamines, lithium, and amitriptyline; it is made worse

FEATURES OF ACTION
PARKINSONIAN AND INTENTION TREMOR

	ACTION (ESSENTIAL)	PARKINSONIAN	INTENTION (CEREBELLAR)
TREMOR IS WORSE:	With sustained posture or contraction	At rest	With projected movement
EXAMINATION:	Normal	Parkinsonian features (rigidity, bradykinesia)	Cerebellar signs
ONSET:	Any age, usually young adulthood	Late in life	Any age
FAMILY HISTORY:	Often present	Absent	May be present
EFFECT OF ALCOHOL:	Usually helps	None	None
FREQUENCY OF TREMOR:	6-11/second	3-7/second	3-5/second
EMG - Agonist / Antagonist			
USEFUL DRUGS:	Propranolol Tranquilizers	Amantadine Anticholinergics L-Dopa Bromocriptine	None

109

by phenothiazines. Remember, tremor may be associated with
Wilson's disease. Treatment: Propranolol (Inderal) 60
mg to 240 mg/day in three or four divided doses is the drug
of choice and is usually effective. Remember, propranolol
may be contraindicated in patients with pulmonary or
cardiac disease. Diazepam (Valium), 10-30 mg/day may also
be of benefit, especially when given in conjunction with
propranolol.

PARKINSON'S DISEASE

The tremor of Parkinson's disease is a gross, 3-7/
second, "pill-rolling" resting tremor which improves with
movement. It occurs in the older patient and is not helped
by alcohol. Examination usually reveals other features of
Parkinsonism: decreased facial expression, rigidity of the
limbs, shuffling gait and slowness in movement (bradykinesia). The patient may also be depressed and, in advanced
stages, suffers from dementia. Parkinson's disease is
secondary to a loss of dopamine in the nigrostriatal pathways. This upsets the normal dopaminergic-cholinergic
balance and the most effective treatment for moderate to
severe Parkinson's disease is exogenous replacement of
L-dopa; anticholinergic medication is also of benefit.

Treatment: There are many regimens for the
treatment of Parkinson's disease. Most clinicians find
that the tremor of Parkinson's disease is helped most by
anticholinergic medication and the akinesia and rigidity
by L-dopa.

1.   Patients with mild Parkinsonism may be treated with
      amantadine (Symmetrel), an anti-viral agent that
      probably benefits Parkinsonian patients by releasing
      dopamine from presynaptic storage sites. A response
      should be seen within a few days. Side effects are
      few and include nausea, visual hallucinations and
      livedo reticularis (a venous mottling of the skin,
      usually around the knees). Livedo reticularis is
      benign and does not require discontinuation of the
      drug.

2.   Anticholinergic medication, e.g., benztropine
      mesylate (Cogentin) or trixyphenidyl (Artane), is
      particularly useful for tremor. Side effects include
      dry mouth, blurred vision and urinary retention.
      Patients with glaucoma should only receive anti-
      cholinergics in conjunction with treatment by an

ophthalmologist. Antihistamines, e.g.,
diphenhydramine (Benadryl), may also be tried and are
weak anti-Parkinsonian agents.

3. L-Dopa is usually given in combination with a
peripheral dopa decarboxylase inhibitor, carbidopa
(Sinemet). Some physicians use L-dopa as the first
drug, particularly in those patients whose
Parkinsonian symptoms interfere in a major way with
their functional status. The decarboxylase inhibitor
increases the amount of L-dopa reaching the CNS.
Thus, it decreases the amount of L-dopa needed and
some of its side effects (e.g., nausea and vomiting)
are avoided. Three strengths of Sinemet in scored
tablets are available: 10/100 mg, 25/100 mg, and
25/250 mg (carbidopa/L-dopa). Patients are usually
begun on 10/100 mg t.i.d. and dosage increased
gradually every other day until the desired
therapeutic effect is reached or side effects occur.
Most patients require 25/250 mg t.i.d. or q.i.d. The
most common side effect of L-dopa therapy is the
development of chorea (involuntary, "jerk-like"
movements that may involve both face and extremities).
In addition, there may be dystonia, agitation,
hallucinations, and paranoia. This "hyperkinesis"
represents the opposite spectrum of the bradykinesia
and akinesia that is characteristic of Parkinsonism
and requires lowering of L-dopa dosage. With lowering
of dosage, Parkinsonian symptoms may recur. At this
stage, administration of small amounts of L-dopa alone
may be of benefit. Amantadine and anticholinergic
drugs can be used concomitantly with L-dopa.
Remember, anticholinergics may slow the absorption of
L-dopa. Amantadine may be effective in patients
receiving L-dopa, even though it did not help when
given alone.

4. Bromocriptine (usual starting dose is 2.5 mg b.i.d.
or t.i.d.), a dopamine agonist, has also been used in
the treatment of Parkinson's disease. It may be
useful in patients with longstanding Parkinson's
disease in whom the effects of L-dopa have worn off.

Note the following:

a. Tricyclic antidepressants can be used for depression in patients receiving L-dopa (they may slow absorption via their anticholinergic effects); monoamine oxidase inhibitors are not recommended.

b. Phenothiazines, haloperidol and reserpine aggravate Parkinsonian symptoms.

c. Pyridoxine antagonizes the effect of L-dopa, but not of Sinemet. Remember, pyridoxine is a vitamin and is often found in vitamin pills.

d. Alpha methyldopa (Aldomet) may potentiate or antagonize the effects of L-dopa.

e. Other side effects of L-dopa (whether given with or without carbidopa) include postural hypotension (usually asymptomatic) and insomnia.

f. The Shy-Drager syndrome is a progressive neurologic disorder consisting of impotence, orthostatic hypotension, plus Parkinsonism due to basal ganglia degeneration. L-dopa is ineffective. Other uncommon neurologic disorders may have symptoms of Parkinsonism, including olivopontocerebellar degeneration, progressive supranuclear palsy, and striatonigral degeneration.

g. Parkinsonism may be secondary to chronic manganese or carbon monoxide intoxication.

h. Physical therapy with a specific list of home exercises is useful in Parkinson's disease. Patients should be encouraged to remain active and mobile.

i. Some patients report a "wearing off" effect of L-dopa, i.e., 2-3 hours after the previous dose. This is treated by giving medication more frequently and/or adding other antiparkinson drugs.

j. The "on-off" effect of L-dopa refers to the sudden loss of the therapeutic effect of L-dopa and can

last minutes to hours. The "on-off" effect is
poorly understood and several treatment regimens
have been tried, e.g., special diets,
discontinuing medication (drug holiday), and use
of drugs such as bromocriptine, lithium, and
monoamine oxidase B inhibitors.

k. Drug-induced Parkinsonism, a toxic effect seen in
patients receiving high doses of neuroleptic drugs
(e.g., phenothiazines), is clinically identical to
idiopathic Parkinsonism. Treatment includes
lowering the dose of the neuroleptic drug plus
anticholinergic medication. Remember, anticholinergics plus phenothiazines potentiate the
appearance of tardive dyskinesia (see below).
L-dopa is contraindicated in drug-induced
Parkinsonism as it usually exacerbates the psycho-
sis. L-dopa induced psychiatric abnormalities are
often benefited by L-tryptophan.

TARDIVE DYSKINESIA

Tardive dyskinesia develops in a significant number
of patients on prolonged treatment with neuroleptic drugs
and often persists after the antipsychotic medication is
discontinued. The drugs most frequently associated with
tardive dyskinesia are the phenothiazines and haloperidol.
Clinically, patients develop an oral-buccal-lingual
dyskinesia (tongue protrusion, lip smacking, facial
grimacing); involuntary movements may involve the limbs
and trunk as well. It is felt that tardive dyskinesia is
caused by an overactivity of brain dopamine associated
with denervation hypersensitivity of brain dopamine
receptors caused by chronic neuroleptic medication. The
main therapeutic approach in tardive dyskinesia is to
deplete brain dopamine with drugs such as reserpine.
Another approach is to use cholinergic agents such as
deanol to modulate the balance between dopamine and
acetylcholine in the striatum. Obviously, elimination or
reduction of neuroleptic therapy should be carried out.
For some patients, tardive dyskinesia is refractory to
medical treatment despite the large number of drugs which
have been employed in this disorder.

OTHER MOVEMENT DISORDERS

1. Hemiballismus, wild, involuntary flinging of an
    extremity, is often secondary to a cerebrovascular
    accident affecting the subthalamic nucleus. There
    also may be hemichorea. Treatment with haloperidol
    (3-8 mg/day) is usually effective, presumably by
    blocking "over-reactive" dopamine receptors in the
    striatum. Some investigators have used perphenazine.

2. Acute dystonic postures (e.g., turning of the neck)
    may occur as an idiosyncratic reaction to neuroleptic
    drugs, e.g., phenothiazines, prochlorperazine
    (Compazine) and usually occurs in young adults. They
    respond dramatically (within minutes) to i.v.
    administration of diphenhydramine (Benadryl) 75 mg, or
    benztropine mesylate (Cogentin) 2 mg. In addition to
    acute dystonia, and drug-induced Parkinsonism
    (discussed previously), neuroleptics can also cause
    akathasia.

3. Myoclonus, or shock-like, non-patterned contraction
    of a portion of a muscle, an entire muscle, or a group
    of muscles occurs in a wide variety of disorders,
    including anoxic brain damage, myoclonic epilepsy, and
    certain degenerative diseases. It can also be seen in
    metabolic encephalopathies and certain drug
    intoxications (e.g., imipramine). Drugs which may be
    useful in treatment include clonazepam, valproic acid,
    and 5-hydroxytryptophan.

REFERENCES

1. Calne DB: Developments in the pharmacology and
    therapeutics of Parkinsonism. Ann Neurol 1: 111,
    1977.
2. Bianchine JR: Drug therapy of Parkinsonism. N Eng J
    Med 295:814, 1976.
3. Fahn S: Management of Parkinson's disease at
    different stages of the illness. Clinical
    Neuropharmacology 5, Suppl. 1, 1982.
4. Jankovic J, Fahn S: Physiologic and pathologic
    tremors. Ann Int Med 93:460-465, 1980.
5. Johnson WG, Fahn S: Treatment of vascular hemiballism
    and hemichoria. Neurology 27:634, 1977.
6. Klawans HL: Tardive dyskinesia: review and update.
    Am J Psych 137:900-908, 1980.

7. Klawans HL, Moses H, Nausieda PA, et al: Treatment and prognosis of hemiballismus. N Eng J Med 295:1348, 1976.

8. Kobayashi RM: Drug therapy of tardive dyskinesia, N Eng J Med 296:257, 1977.

9. Marsden CD, Parkes JD: Success and problems of long-term levodopa therapy in Parkinson's disease. Lancet 1:345, 1977.

10. Moskowitz MA, Wurtman RJ: Catecholamines and neurologic diseases. N Eng J Med 293:274, 1975.

11. Van Woert MH, Rosenbaum D, Howieson J, Bowers MB: Long-term therapy of myoclonus and other neurologic disorders with L-5-hydroxytryptophan and carbidopa. N Eng J Med 296:70, 1977.

12. Winkler GF, Young RR: Efficacy of chronic propranolol therapy in action tremors of the familial, senile or essential varities. N Eng J Med 290:984, 1974.

13. Lewitt PA, Chase TN: "On-off" effects: the new challenge in Parkinsonism. Trends in Neurosciences 6:1, 1983.

Chapter 18

Ataxia

Ataxia is a disorder of coordination and rhythm. Because there are many parts of the nervous system that participate in carrying out coordinated movements, ataxia may result from anatomic dysfunction at different levels of the neuraxis. The best way to establish the cause of ataxia is to determine what level of the nervous system is involved. In this chapter, ataxia is classified anatomically and some of the common causes of ataxia are discussed.

IS THE LESION IN THE <u>FRONTAL LOBE</u>? (Mechanism: involvement of cortico-cerebellar connections, i.e., fronto-ponto-cerebellar pathway).

1. <u>Tumor</u>. Meningioma, glioma, or metastatic tumor may involve the frontal lobes. Patients may have signs of cerebellar disease, i.e., staggering gait, difficulty performing rapid alternating movements, and even nystagmus, although these signs are present in only about half of patients with frontal lobe tumors. Patients with "frontal ataxia" tend to fall backwards. Other features of frontal lobe dysfunction include perseveration, grasp and suck reflexes, incontinence, and slowness in mentation. There is often headache and patients may be demented (see Chapter 21). Diagnosis is via CAT scan.

2. <u>Anterior cerebral artery syndrome</u>. A thrombotic occlusion of this artery affects the frontal lobes (see Chapter 6). A large aneurysm of the anterior communicating artery may also affect the frontal lobes.

3.   **Hydrocephalus**. Enlargement of the frontal horns of
the lateral ventricles affects leg fibers and may
produce ataxia. In addition, there is memory loss
and incontinence. Hydrocephalus may occur with
tumors that obstruct the ventricular system or with
more diffuse problems of CSF absorption (e.g., normal
pressure hydrocephalus, see Chapter 10).

IS THE LESION **SUBCORTICAL**? (Mechanism: involvement of
cortico-cerebellar connections plus pyramidal tract
dysfunction).

1.   **Multiple strokes** (état lacunaire). In addition to
ataxia, there is emotional lability, brisk reflexes,
including increased jaw jerk, dysarthria, and
dementia (see Chapter 10).

IN THE **BRAINSTEM**? (Mechanism: involvement of
cerebellar tracts).

1.   The two most common causes of ataxia secondary to
brainstem lesions are cerebrovascular accidents and
multiple sclerosis. Diagnosis is based on history
and finding other brainstem signs (e.g., crossed
motor or sensory findings, internuclear
ophthalmoplegia, nystagmus, dysarthria).

IS THE LESION IN THE **CEREBELLUM**? (Mechanism: direct
involvement of coordination pathway).

1.   **Signs** of cerebellar dysfunction include limb,
trunk, gait and speech ataxia, nystagmus, and
hypotonia. Depending on whether midline or lateral
cerebellar structures are involved, there may or may
not be limb ataxia or prominent lateral gaze
nystagmus. Midline lesions tend to produce truncal
and gait ataxia, whereas hemisphere lesions primarily
produce limb ataxia.

2.   **Cerebellar hemorrhage, infarct, tumor**. There are
often occipital headache and ocular gaze palsies.
Limb strength and sensation are preserved.
Cerebellar hemorrhage is an acute process requiring
immediate diagnosis (CAT scan) and usually surgical
intervention (see Chapter 6). Primary cerebellar
tumors are seen in childhood, they are rare in
adults; metastatic tumors involve the cerebellum in
adults.

3. Spinocerebellar degeneration. These syndromes
    include olivo-ponto-cerebellar degeneration and
    Freidreich's ataxia. There is usually a positive
    family history and evidence of widespread nervous
    system involvement, e.g., peripheral neuropathy (loss
    of reflexes), pyramidal tract dysfunction (upgoing
    toes). Pes cavus or scoliosis are associated with
    some of these entities.

4. Alcoholism or occult malignancy may be associated
    with cerebellar degeneration. Alcoholic cerebellar
    degeneration is characterized by ataxia of gait and
    of the legs, with less prominent involvement of arms,
    speech, or ocular motility. There is usually an
    associated polyneuropathy. Acute ataxia and
    oculomotor paralysis associated with alcoholism
    (Wernicke's encephalopathy) responds to thiamine
    administration (see Chapter 23). Remember,
    cerebellar ataxia as a "remote" effect may be the
    presenting symptoms of an occult malignancy (see
    Chapter 21).

IS THE LESION IN THE SPINAL CORD? (Mechanism: ataxia
via posterior column dysfunction, involvement of
spinocerebellar tracts, or spasticity from involvement of
pyramidal tracts). Remember, a positive Romberg sign
(unsteady with eyes closed, steady with eyes open) usually
indicates posterior column disease.

1. Cervical spondylosis with associated cervical
    myelopathy. Patients usually have neck and arm pain
    and abnormal cervical spine films. Depending on the
    extent of spinal cord involvement, there may be
    posterior column dysfunction and upgoing toes
    (pyramidal tract involvement).

2. Multiple sclerosis often involves the spinal cord.
    Diagnosis is made on the basis of finding multiple
    lesions of the nervous system (e.g., optic neuritis,
    brainstem signs) and a history of prior attacks.
    Usually, there is elevation of CSF gamma globulin.

3. Vitamin B_{12} deficiency may produce combined system
    disease, i.e., involvement of posterior and lateral
    columns of the spinal cord. Patients first notice
    generalized weakness and paresthesias. Later, there
    is leg stiffness and ataxia. Loss of vibration and
    position sense occurs, associated with upgoing toes

and often, diminished or absent knee and ankle jerks secondary to peripheral neuropathy. There may be mental changes (see Chapter 10).

4. **Syringomyelia** is a chronic, progressive disorder of spinal cord and at times, medulla (syringobulbia). Cavitation within the substance of the spinal cord causes sensory dissociation (pain and temperature loss with preservation of touch and position sense), anterior horn cell involvement (muscle wasting fasciculations, absent reflexes in the upper extremities) cortico-spinal tract involvement (spasticity), and trophic disorders secondary to involvement of spinal sympathetic fibers. Patients often have scoliosis. Syringomyelia may be congenital or acquired (e.g., post-traumatic).

5. Other causes of ataxia secondary to spinal cord dysfunction include spinal cord tumor, spinocerebellar degeneration, tabes dorsalis, and amyotrophic lateral sclerosis.

IS THE LESION IN <u>PERIPHERAL NERVE</u>? (Mechanism: ataxia secondary to weakness and, in idiopathic polyneuritis, due to dorsal root involvement)

1. Idiopathic polyneuritis (Guillain-Barré). The Guillain-Barré syndrome may present as ataxia in its early stages or, if the polyneuritis is mild, be its major clinical manifestation. Diagnosis is based on absent reflexes, increased CSF protein, and slowed nerve conduction times (see Chapter 15). Ataxia may also be a feature of severe peripheral neuropathies from other causes.

IS THE LESION IN <u>MUSCLE</u>? (Mechanism: ataxia secondary to muscle weakness)

1. **Myopathy**, whether acquired (e.g., polymyositis, thyroid myopathy) or congenital (muscular dystrophy), may be associated with ataxia. Diagnosis is made on the basis of physical examination, muscle enzymes and muscle biopsy (see Chapter 16).

Rarer causes of <u>chronic progressive ataxia</u> include Charcot-Marie-Tooth disease, Ramsey Hunt syndrome, familial spastic ataxia and Huntington's chorea. Ataxia may be associated with Refsum's syndrome,

abetalipoproteinemia, juvenile dystonic lipidosis, and may
be seen in meningeal leukemia or in association with
occult neuroblastoma and hypothyroidism.

Acute forms have been associated with drug and
chemical ingestion (e.g., alcohol, lead), acute
labyrinthitis, post-ictal states, sickle cell crisis, and
lupus erythematosis. The rapidity of onset, other
clinical features, and lab findings usually permit rapid
differentiation of acute ataxia from the chronic forms.

In addition to a careful history and physical
examination, the CAT scan has proved invaluable in the
diagnosis of ataxia secondary to cerebellar infarct or
hemorrhage, cerebellar or frontal lobe tumor, and normal
pressure hydrocephalus. Other studies, such as CSF gamma
globulin in multiple sclerosis, B_{12} level in pernicious
anemia, and cervical spine films for cervical spondylosis,
are obtained when these diagnoses are suspected on
clinical grounds.

Chapter 19

Peripheral Nerve and Root Dysfunction

To diagnose peripheral nerve and root injuries, one must determine which muscles are affected and the territory of the sensory loss. Thus, one must know which roots and nerves supply which muscles and their sensory distribution.

REFLEXES

Reflexes are diminished in root and peripheral nerve disease. (Root irritation alone or damage to a root not involved in the reflex arc does not decrease the reflex.) There are four primary reflexes to remember, with particular roots and muscles necessary for their function. An easy way to learn the roots is to remember that, going from ankle to triceps, the roots are numbered consecutively from one to eight.

THE FOUR PRIMARY REFLEXES

Reflex	Roots needed for reflex	Muscle carrying out the reflex
Ankle jerk	S1	Gastrocnemius
Knee jerk	L2, L3, L4	Quadriceps
Biceps	C5, C6	Biceps
Triceps	C7, C8	Triceps

ROOTS AND MUSCLES

There is an overlap between roots and the muscles they supply; thus, more than one root is generally responsible for each muscle. Nevertheless, certain muscles serve as standard clinical indices for each root so that if one particular root is out, there should be one muscle (or muscle group) that is particularly weak.

Each root has a sensory distribution as represented on the standard dermatome chart (see Chapter 28).

Roots and the Primary Muscles They Supply

Root	Muscle	Action
C5	Deltoid	Shoulder abduction
C5	Infraspinatus	Humeral external rotation (check: have patient externally rotate the humerus with the arm held at side and flexed at the elbow, as if shooting a gun)

(Continued on following page)

Roots and the Primary Muscles They Supply (cont'd.)

Root	Muscle	Action
C5,C6	Biceps	Flexion of the supinated forearm
C6	Extensor carpi radialis and ulnaris	Wrist extension
C7	Extensors digitorum Triceps	Finger extension; forearm extension at elbow
C8,T1	Interossei and lumbricals	Digital abduction and adduction (check: have patient move fingers apart and together against resistance)
L2,L3,L4	Quadriceps Iliopsoas Adductor group	Knee extension Thigh on hip flexion Thigh adduction
L5	Anterior tibial and extensor hallucis	Ankle and large toe dorsiflexion (check: have patient walk on heels)
S1	Gastrocnemius	Ankle plantar flexion (check: have patient walk on tiptoes)

CHARACTERISTIC FEATURES
ASSOCIATED WITH VARIOUS NERVES

Nerve	Involvement
Median	Thumb and thenar eminence
Ulnar	Little finger and hypothenar eminence
Radial	Wrist-drop
Femoral	Absent knee jerk (weak hip flexion and knee extension)
Peroneal	Foot-drop
Sciatic	Pain down lateral thigh and leg, often with absent ankle jerk

NERVES AND MUSCLES OF
THE UPPER EXTREMITY

Median Nerve

The median nerve (C6-T1) originates in the shoulder (brachial plexus) and supplies two basic muscle groups:

. Forearm: pronator of the forearm, radial flexion, and wrist abduction.

. Hand: first two Lumbricales (index and middle finger flexion at the metacarpal-phalangeal joint); thumb Opposition, Abduction, and Flexion. ("LOAF" muscles.)

Sensory loss involves the thumb, index, middle, and half of the ring finger.

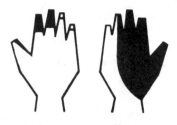

Clinical comment: A complete median nerve lesion (both forearm and hand muscles) is usually secondary to traumatic injury in the axilla or a lesion affecting the median nerve at the elbow. Partial involvement (at the wrist) is one of the most frequently encountered mononeuropathies and is termed the carpal tunnel syndrome (as median nerve is compressed in carpal tunnel). Patients will often complain of numbness and tingling in the thumb and first two fingers; muscle wasting and loss of power (thenar eminence) occur later. The diagnosis may be confirmed by nerve conduction studies. The carpal tunnel syndrome is often bilateral and may be associated with systemic processes; look for rheumatoid arthritis, myxedema, diabetes, pregnancy, gout, acromegaly, and amyloidosis. Medical management includes treating the underlying disease, administering diuretics, splinting the wrist, and injection of steroids into the carpal tunnel. Surgical decompression of the carpal tunnel may be necessary and is usually successful.

// When median nerve involvement is suspected, think of thumb and thenar eminence//

Ulnar Nerve

The ulnar nerve (C8-Tl) is the counterpart of the median nerve in the forearm and hand. It supplies all muscles and sensory areas (on palm) not supplied by the median nerve. When ulnar nerve disease is suspected, think of little finger and hypothenar eminence. The ulnar nerve runs in the ulnar groove at the medial aspect of the elbow ("funny bone") and supplies the following two muscle groups:

. <u>Forearm</u>: ulnar flexion at the wrist

. <u>Hand</u>: little finger abduction and opposition,
thumb adduction, all the interosseous muscles
(used to spread fingers apart and bring together);
third and fourth lumbricales (ring and little
finger flexion at the metacarpal-phalangeal joint)

<u>Sensory loss</u> involves the fourth and little finger.

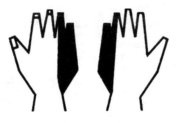

     <u>Clinical comment</u>: Ulnar nerve palsy gives a "claw
hand" deformity with extension of the ring and little
fingers (ability to flex is lost). The ulnar nerve is
commonly injured at the elbow where it is most exposed.
Tardive (or delayed) ulnar palsy may occur years after
trauma to the elbow (perhaps when fibrosis becomes
significant). Look for muscle weakness as opposed to the
prominent sensory symptoms seen in median nerve
dysfunction. A claw hand is also seen with involvement of
C8-Tl roots at the origin of the brachial plexus due to
trauma, surgery, or tumor at the apex of the lung. Check
for Horner's syndrome (small pupil and ptosis) on the same
side as the claw hand. This indicates sympathetic fiber
involvement in the area of the brachial plexus.

<u>Radial Nerve</u>

     The radial nerve (C5-C8) winds around the lateral
aspect of the elbow. When one suspects radial nerve
involvement, think of wrist-drop.

The radial nerve supplies these muscles:

. <u>Supinator</u> of the forearm

. <u>Extensors</u> of the fingers, wrist, elbow (triceps), and of the thumb

<u>Sensory loss</u> involves the back of the hand and is not always present.

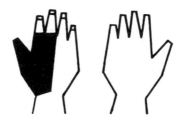

<u>Clinical comment</u>: Injury to the radial nerve may occur in the axilla (e.g., after using crutches) giving inability to extend the elbow plus wrist-drop. If the radial nerve is involved at the elbow, only wrist-drop is found. Pressure palsies are common ("Saturday night palsy" and "bridegroom's palsy", where groom sleeps with bride's head on his arm). In addition, the radial nerve is affected in diabetes and lead poisoning. In radial nerve palsy, ability to spread fingers apart (ulnar nerve function) may be weak due to the mechanical disadvantage caused by the wrist-drop. Check with wrist resting on a flat surface (e.g., table) to overcome that handicap.

Cervical Discs

Herniated discs causing nerve root compression are less common in the cervical than in the lumbar area. They should be suspected when a patient's sensory findings and/or symptoms conform to a particular root distribution and are accompanied by reflex and motor dysfunction of the same root. Note associated neck pain.

Cervical Spondylosis

Check for (1) multiple, often asymmetrical root involvement in the upper extremities, with muscle wasting and hypoactive reflexes in the distribution of those roots affected; (2) compression of the cervical spinal cord giving hyperactive lower extremity reflexes, upgoing toes, and later, leg weakness. Remember, sensory symptoms in the hands plus spastic lower extremities in patients over 50 equals cervical spondylosis with myelopathy until proven otherwise (check B_{12} level). Similar symptoms may be caused by foramen magnum tumors, especially in younger patients.

NERVES AND MUSCLES OF
THE LOWER EXTREMITY

The <u>obturator nerve</u> (L2-L3-L4 roots, ventral portion) supplies the adductors of the thigh. It may be damaged during labor, involved in diabetes, or affected by local pelvic disease.

Femoral Nerve

The <u>femoral nerve</u> (L2-L3-L4 roots, dorsal portion) supplies the iliopsoas (hip flexion) and quadriceps (knee extension). The knee jerk is diminished or absent. Femoral nerve involvement may be distinguished from root involvement at L2-L3-L4 (e.g., by paravertebral tumor) by checking thigh adduction (obturator), which is affected if roots are involved but spared if the femoral nerve alone is involved. <u>Causes</u> of femoral neuropathy include diabetes (look for quadriceps wasting with pain over the anterior thigh), tumor, polyarteritis, and pelvic trauma.

Lateral Femoral Cutaneous Nerve

This pure sensory nerve (L2-L3) supplies the lateral thigh. There is tingling, burning and pain. The lateral femoral cutaneous nerve syndrome (meralgia paresthetica) is common in diabetes, appears during pregnancy or as a result of pressure from a corset, a tight fitting belt, obesity, or even poor posture. Treatment involves removing the offending agent, and, if necessary, injection of the nerve at its entrance to the thigh with xylocaine and steroids, or surgical transection.

Sciatic Nerve

The sciatic nerve (L4-S3) supplies hamstrings (flexion of the knee) and all muscles below the knee.

At the knee it divides into the:

- . Peroneal, which runs anteriorly and supplies muscles that dorsiflex and evert the foot and sensation on top of the foot.

- . Posterior tibial, which runs posteriorly at the knee and supplies muscles of plantar flexion and inversion and sensation on the sole of the foot.

Clinically, the most common affliction of the sciatic nerve is sciatica, a painful sensory disturbance beginning in the buttock and moving down the lateral aspect of the thigh. Irritation of any root from L4-S3 may produce sciatica to a varying degree. One of the most common causes of sciatica is lumbar disc protrusion (pain may be precipitated by coughing or sneezing), often with associated reflex loss and weakness in a root distribution. Straight leg raising generally aggravates the back pain. In some patients there may be no neurologic findings with a herniated disc, although often there is paravertebral muscle spasm.

Most Common Lumbar Disc Syndromes

Root	Disc Interspace	Reflex affected	Motor weakness	Sensory changes (if any)
L4	L3-L4	Knee jerk	Knee extension	Anterior thigh
L5	L4-Sl	Posterior tibial may be helpful	Large toe dorsi-flexion	Large toe
Sl	L5-Sl	Ankle jerk	Foot, plantar flexion	Foot, lateral border

The decision to carry out myelography, CAT scan, and/or surgery for lumbar disc disease depends on the ability to relieve pain with bed rest (10-14 days of complete bedrest is usually necessary) and physical therapy and the presence of weakness or other abnormal neurologic signs. Some have advocated short courses of high dose dexamethasone for disc disease.

Peroneal Nerve

The peroneal nerve supplies dorsiflexors (tibialis anterior) and everters (turning out) of the foot. Inverters (turning in of foot) are supplied by the posterior tibial nerve. The sensory distribution involves the lateral aspect of the leg and dorsum of the foot.

Clinically, peroneal nerve palsy gives foot-drop and is analogous to wrist-drop (radial nerve) in the upper extremity. Foot-drop is seen in diabetics and is a frequent pressure palsy (due to the superficial location of the nerve at the lateral aspect of the knee) -- either from trauma or pressure in a thin or wasted individual. Hereditary peroneal neuropathy (Charcot-Marie-Tooth disease) is associated with bilateral foot-drop, a wasted anterior leg compartment below the knee, and pes cavus. Remember, peroneal palsy spares the inverters of the foot; if they too are weak, the lesion is higher, generally at the root, sciatic nerve, or cord level.

Posterior Tibial Nerve

This nerve is rarely injured alone, as it runs deep in the calf.

CONUS MEDULLARIS AND CAUDA EQUINA LESIONS

The conus medullaris (lower sacral segments of the spinal cord) and cauda equina (elongated roots of the lumbar and sacral spinal nerves) can each be affected by a variety of processes. Helpful distinguishing features between lesions of the conus and cauda equina are contained in the following table:

	Conus Medullaris	Cauda Equina
Motor weakness	Absent or mild	Present and unilateral
Sensory deficits	Bilateral (saddle)	Unilateral
Sphincter involvement	Early; of bladder and bowel	Late and mild
Differential diagnoses	Tumor, hemorrhage disk, pelvic fracture, spondylolisthesis	Same

INVESTIGATION OF NERVE AND ROOT DYSFUNCTION

Examine the patient to determine whether the nerve or root is involved. Determine whether the sensory loss (or symptom) and muscle weakness (if present) fit the distribution of a particular nerve or root.

Establish the _etiology_. If a particular nerve or root is definitely involved, determine the specific etiologic factors unique to that nerve or root. Important to ask:

1. Did a nerve palsy come on after _sleep_ or _surgery_ (pressure palsies)?

2. Is there evidence of _trauma_, old or new?

3. What are the patient's _occupation_ and habits? For example, there may be median nerve involvement in gardeners and beauty operators, ulnar nerve damage in cornhuskers.

4. Is there evidence of _systemic disease_ (e.g., diabetes, breast cancer affecting the brachial plexus, or polyarteritis)?

TRIGEMINAL NEURALGIA (Tic Douloureux)

Excruciating, paroxysmal pain lasting seconds to minutes in the distribution of the second or third division of the fifth cranial nerve is the hallmark of trigeminal neuralgia. The pain is often "triggered" by touching the side of the face or brought on by facial movement such as chewing. There is no objective motor or sensory loss. The cause is unknown but may be related to a viral infection or to pressure on the nerve by a basilar artery branch near the brainstem. Trigeminal neuralgia is uncommon in people under 40 and when it occurs in the younger patient, particularly if associated with objective sensory loss, it is frequently secondary to multiple sclerosis. The presence of neurologic signs (loss of sensation on the face, cranial nerve palsies, long tract signs) suggests focal pathology such as tumor, vascular malformation or demyelinating disease. Treatment with carbamazepine (Tegretol) relieves pain in the majority of patients (begin with 100 mg b.i.d., increase by 100 mg/day up to 1200 mg/day; monitor hematologic indices). Patients refractory to medical treatment require surgical intervention; percutaneous radiofrequency coagulation of the Gasserian ganglion may be extremely effective in relieving the pain of trigeminal neuralgia and some patients have had vascular compression of the trigeminal nerve relieved via craniotomy.

SEVENTH NERVE PALSIES, INCLUDING BELL'S PALSY

Peripheral involvement of the 7th cranial nerve is a well recognized syndrome. Onset may be heralded by pain behind the ear and diagnosis is based on demonstrating complete facial palsy, i.e., paralysis of both lower face and forehead, in the absence of other neurologic findings. Central lesions which affect fibers prior to their synapse in the 7th nerve nucleus in the brainstem spare forehead musculature. In addition to innervating facial musculature, fibers from the 7th nerve innervate the lacrimal gland of the eye, the stapedius muscle in the ear (hyperacusis), the submaxillary and sublingual glands, and carry afferent taste fibers from the anterior two-thirds of the tongue. The majority of cases are idiopathic (Bell's palsy). Other causes include infectious mononucleosis, the Guillain-Barré syndrome (bilateral 7th nerve palsies, loss of reflexes, see p. 98), fracture, severe hypertension, diabetes, sarcoid and histiocytosis, and an associated otitis or mastoiditis. A cerebellopontine angle tumor or a brainstem plaque from multiple sclerosis may give a peripheral 7th nerve palsy, usually in association with other cranial nerve signs. Melkersson's syndrome is recurrent 7th nerve palsies associated with facial edema.

Treatment with prednisone probably hastens recovery and the amount of residual facial dysfiguration in the idiopathic (Bell's palsy) variety and should be given within the first 72 hours of onset: 60 mg daily for four days, then taper to 5 mg/day in ten days. Patching the eye and methylcellulose eye drops will help prevent corneal ulceration. Surgical decompression probably is of no benefit. Recovery usually begins within one to four weeks of onset and may take longer than three months to be complete. Patients with hyperacusis, taste loss or defective tearing have a poorer prognosis (proximal lesion of the facial nerve). Remember to perform a careful neurologic exam in search of other neurologic signs in patients with a peripheral 7th nerve palsy.

THORACIC OUTLET SYNDROME

The thoracic outlet syndrome refers to symptoms and signs which occur due to compression of the subclavian vessels and brachial plexus at the superior aperture of the thorax between the first rib and the clavicle. Symptoms include pain and paresthesias in the neck, shoulder, arm, and hand (C8, T1 distribution), weakness of the hand, change of color of the hand, including pallor of the fingers, and aggravation of all symptoms by use of the upper limb. Signs depend on whether primarily vascular or neural compression exists and include supraclavicular bruit, loss or diminution of radial pulse, weakness and sensory loss in the hand and reproduction of pain by traction on the arm. Anomalies of the spine are often present, including cervical ribs or abnormal transverse process of C7.

REFERENCES

1.   Adour KK: Diagnosis and management of facial paralysis. N Engl J Med 307:348, 1982.
2.   Aids to the Investigation of Peripheral Nerve Injuries. London, Her Majesty's Stationery Office, 1976.

3.   Green LN: Dexamethasone in the management of symptoms
     due to herniated lumbar disk. _J Neurol Neurosurg
     Psych_ 38:1211, 1975.
4.   Haymaker W, Woodhall B: _Peripheral Nerve Injuries_.
     Philadelphia, W.B. Saunders, 1967.
5.   Kopell HP, Thompson WA: _Peripheral entrapment
     neuropathies_. Krieger, 1976.
6.   Lascelles RG, et al.: The thoracic outlet syndrome.
     Brain 100:601, 1977.
7.   Liveson JA, Spielholz NI: _Peripheral Neurology Case
     Studies in Electrodiagnosis_. FA Davis, 1979.
8.   Sunderland S: _Nerves and Nerve Injuries_. London,
     Churchill-Livingstone, 1972.

Chapter 20

Neurology of Diabetes

Diabetes frequently manifests a variety of neurologic symptoms; indeed, "neuropathy" is a classic diabetic complication. Most of the neurological complications of diabetes are not referable to the central nervous system. Cerebrovascular disease, although more common in diabetes, is not a diabetic phenomenon -- but one to which the diabetic is prone.

DIABETIC "NEUROPATHY"

Polyneuropathy

Polyneuropathy is the most common diabetic neuropathy; it manifests as a symmetrical, distal ("glove and stocking") sensory polyneuropathy, sparing motor function. The upper border of the sensory loss is irregular; ankle jerks are generally absent and vibration sense is diminished. This benign neuropathy usually does not bring the patient to the physician and, apart from minor paresthesias, is asymptomatic. It can, however, lead to trophic changes and injury from trauma because of the loss of pain sensation.

Mononeuropathy

Mononeuropathy is a dramatic diabetic neuropathy that probably results from nerve infarction. The onset of motor and sensory loss in one nerve is abrupt and often painful; the involved nerve may be tender. Prognosis is good and recovery usually occurs in four to six months.

Treatment is with physical therapy and appropriate support (splints where needed).

There is a predilection for certain nerves. The most commonly affected are:

1.   <u>Oculomotor (III) nerve</u>. The patient has diplopia and may have pain over the eye. There is an almost total ophthalmoplegia (lateral eye movement is spared). The clue to a "diabetic third" is that the pupillary fibers are usually spared. (The pupillary fibers are on the outer perimeter of the nerve, and vascular infarction occurs centrally.) Thus, the pupil is of normal size and reacts -- it is not large and unreactive as in other third nerve palsies (e.g., those due to compression).

2.   <u>Abducens (VI) nerve</u>. There is an isolated inability to move the eye laterally. Remember, a sixth nerve palsy may also be the first sign of increased intracranial pressure (check for headache and papilledema).

3.   <u>Femoral nerve</u>. There is pain in the lateral and anterior thigh; weakness and atrophy of quadriceps (extension at knee) plus weakness of iliopsoas (flexion of hip); and a diminished or absent knee jerk (see Chapter 19).

4.   <u>Radial nerve and peroneal nerve</u>. There is wrist-drop or foot-drop (see Chapter 19).

5.   <u>Facial (VII) nerve</u>. Bell's palsy is more common in diabetics (see Chapter 19).

Radiculopathy

<u>Radiculopathy</u> is secondary to involvement of the posterior root outside the spinal cord before it becomes a mixed nerve. Clinically, the patient complains of shooting pains often confined to one dermatome. There are usually no motor or reflex changes. This neuropathy may be difficult to distinguish from disc disease and fortunately resolves spontaneously. Lumbar and thoracic roots are most frequently affected, and involvement may be bilateral. Sometimes there is posterior column degeneration, resulting in posterior column dysfunction and shooting pains. If the patient has these symptoms plus an irregular pupil that accommodates but reacts

poorly to light (sometimes seen in diabetics), the term
"diabetic pseudotabes" is used.

Amyotrophy

Amyotrophy is generally seen in older patients and
consists of pain in the thighs and proximal muscle
weakness and wasting. Quadriceps and hamstrings may also
be weak, and the patient complains of myalgia and
dysesthesias in the thighs, although there is no objective
sensory loss. Knee and ankle reflexes are usually absent,
and toes may be upgoing. There is evidence to indicate
that amyotrophy is a neuropathic process with proximal
motor nerves of the lower extremities being affected
preferentially. The prognosis is good, with recovery
occurring over 6 to 12 months, particularly with optimum
control of the diabetes. (Check for other causes of
proximal muscle weakness -- e.g., endocrine myopathy,
polymyositis.)

Autonomic Neuropathy

The most common manifestations of autonomic
neuropathy are orthostatic hypotension (treat with
elastic stockings, mineralocorticoids), nocturnal
diarrhea, impotence, urinary retention, and abdominal
distension.

COMMENTS ON DIABETES
AND THE NERVOUS SYSTEM

There is no specific treatment for the various
diabetic neuropathies. The physician should make sure
that the neuropathies are associated with diabetes and do
not represent symptoms due to other treatable processes.
Support and physical therapy are important during the
period of recovery. There is some evidence that
neuropathies may be ameliorated by careful medical
management of the diabetic. Drugs such as amytriptyline
or phenytoin may be useful for the pain or paresthesias of
diabetic neuropathy.

// CSF protein is
frequently elevated in
diabetes //

Remember, spinal fluid protein is frequently
elevated in diabetes.

Diabetic coma and hypoglycemia are not discussed in detail here.   Remember to draw a blood sugar and administer 50% glucose intravenously to all patients presenting with coma of uncertain cause.   Patients with hypoglycemia may present with behavioral disturbances, seizures, and even focal neurologic deficits that clear with glucose administration.   Treatment of hyperglycemia and coma may result in hypokalemia and a flaccid paralysis.

Diabetics are at increased risk for cerebrovascular disease.

Cervical spondylosis is more apt to be symptomatic in the diabetic than the nondiabetic.   There may be hyperactive reflexes at the knees with upgoing toes (secondary to compression of the cord at the cervical region), and loss of ankle jerks and vibration sense (secondary to the diabetic neuropathy).

REFERENCES

1.   Asbury AK: Proximal diabetic neuropathy. Ann Neurol 2:179, 1977.
2.   Asbury AK, Aldredge H, Hershberg R, et al.: Oculomotor palsy in diabetes mellitus: A clinico-pathological study. Brain 93:555, 1970.
3.   Bastron JA, Thomas JE: Diabetic polyradiculopathy: Clinical and electromyographic findings in 105 patients. Mayo Clin Proc 56:725, 1981.
4.   Kozak GP, et al.: Diabetic neuropathies. Am Fam Phys 15:112, 122, 1977.
5.   Raff MC, Asbury AK: Ischemic mononeuropathy and mononeuropathy multiplex in diabetes mellitus. N Engl J Med 279:17, 1968.
6.   Spritz N: Nerve disease in diabetes mellitus. Med Clin N Am 62(4):787, July 1978.

Chapter 21

Malignancy and the Nervous System

Malignancy may affect the nervous system in two ways: 1) By direct involvement of either primary or metastatic brain or spinal cord tumor; and 2) By non-metastatic effects, when nervous system dysfunction is associated with malignancy elsewhere in the body.

SIGNS AND SYMPTOMS OF BRAIN TUMOR

These signs and symptoms apply to both primary and metastatic CNS tumors.

1. Does the patient have <u>headache</u>? This is one of the most common symptoms, being present in about two-thirds of patients. It is often present in the morning.

2. Other signs and symptoms include seizures, personality changes, hemiplegia, and visual disturbances. Mental changes, especially memory loss and decreased alertness are often important subtle clues of intracranial tumor.

3. Patients may have a <u>gait disturbance</u>.

4. <u>Seizures</u> associated with tumor are characteristically focal. They may be Jacksonian: a focal seizure that begins in one extremity and then "marches" until it becomes a generalized convulsion.

5. Check for <u>papilledema</u> or sixth nerve paresis due to raised intracranial pressure.

6.   Sometimes there may be bleeding within a tumor or
      vessel occlusion, creating the clinical picture of a
      cerebrovascular accident.   Some tumors have a
      propensity to bleed (e.g., melanoma).

INTRACRANIAL METASTASES

Which Tumors Invade the Brain?

Metastatic tumor reaches the brain via hematogenous
spread and generally after first invading the lung.   This
accounts for the high incidence of intracranial metastases
with lung and breast tumor.   Tumors of the
gastrointestinal tract may metastasize to the brain,
although they do so less frequently and generally invade
the liver and lung first.   Hypernephroma and melanoma
are important sources of CNS metastases but are less
common tumors.   Prostatic carcinoma, a common tumor in
elderly men, very rarely goes

// Prostatic cancer rarely
metastasizes to the brain //

to the brain.   Theoretically, metastases might occur via
Batson's venous plexus near the lower spinal cord, but the
rarity of prostatic metastases to brain demonstrates how
nonfunctional this route actually is.   Tumors of the
cervix and ovary also metastasize to the brain
infrequently.

When Do Tumors Metastasize
to the Brain?

The majority of metastases occur within two years of
discovery of the primary lesion, although they can
sometimes appear years after the removal of a primary
source (e.g., with kidney or breast cancer).   Conversely,
a metastatic tumor may be the first sign of a primary
neoplasm elsewhere, especially lung cancer.

When a neurologic symptom (e.g., seizure) is
secondary to a brain metastasis, obvious neurological
progression will usually occur within six months.   For
example, a patient with known breast carcinoma who has a
convulsion and then remains neurologically intact for a
year probably did not experience the seizure because of
a cerebral metastasis.

Laboratory Investigation

1. Brain scan and EEG are usually abnormal in patients with brain tumor; CAT scan is the most reliable test and should be done with contrast if the non-contrast CAT scan is normal. An LP should not be performed if an intracranial tumor is suspected (see Chapter 26).

2. Arteriography may be necessary to confirm the diagnosis and help in distinguishing primary from metastatic lesions. Brain biopsy as a method of diagnosis carries a considerable risk in mortality and morbidity.

3. The physician must evaluate each patient individually in terms of which studies to perform.

Treatment

The treatment of primary brain tumor depends on the tumor type and location. Meningiomas are usually removable. Low grade astrocytomas and oligodendrogliomas are best treated by surgery plus irradiation. High grade astrocytomas (glioblastoma multiforme) are treated by biopsy plus irradiation or, depending on location, partial removal plus irradiation. The role of chemotherapy is controversial, but it is probably useful.

In the approach to patients with metastatic brain tumor, one must first determine whether the brain is involved by single or multiple metastases. Documented multiple metastases are treated with steroids and whole brain irradiation. Symptoms are ameliorated with steroids (reduction of cerebral edema). Irradiation improves both length and quality of survival. Chemotherapy may be added. Treatment of a single metastasis is controversial. Some authors advocate surgical removal; in addition to offering palliation, other processes are sometimes found at operation (e.g., subdural hematoma, primary brain tumor). Nevertheless, the associated risks of craniotomy are real, and often there are multiple metastases that were not revealed by laboratory investigation. Nuclear magnetic resonance (NMR) may allow a more precise diagnosis of multiple metastases, making this decision easier.

The choice of treatment (surgery, steroids, or irradiation) for the patient with a single metastasis depends on the extent and nature of his primary tumor, his individual circumstances (e.g., age and medical condition), and the philosophy of his primary physician, and neurologist or neurosurgeon.

METASTATIC TUMOR TO THE SPINAL CORD

Management

Metastatic tumor to the cord (generally epidural implant) may compress the cord and constitutes a neurologic emergency. Carcinoma of the lung, breast or prostate, or lymphomas and leukemias may cause spinal cord compression. Back pain, tenderness, change in urinary frequency, or symptoms of root involvement often appear prior to compression. Plain films of the spine usually are abnormal, except with lymphoma. See Chapter 14 for evaluation and treatment of acute spinal cord compression.

LEUKEMIA AND LYMPHOMA

These malignant processes are frequently associated with nervous system dysfunction, although they usually do not invade the brain and spinal cord. With more effective treatment and with patients living longer, there has been an increasing incidence of CNS complications.

Leukemia

Leukemia is associated with a triad of neurologic complications.

1. **Intracranial hemorrhage** is common in leukemia (often fatal) and is usually related to a low platelet count or a high leukocyte count (greater than 100,000 per mm). Intracranial bleeding occurs in multiple areas (not usually one, as in hypertensive bleeding) and is often associated with systemic bleeding. Once bleeding has occurred, transfusion therapy is of little benefit. Therefore, maintaining hematologic indices as normal as possible before neurologic complications occur is crucial.

2. **Leukemic infiltration** of meninges (both of brain and spinal cord) and nerve roots is common and frequently occurs when the patient is in hematologic remission. Meningeal leukemia usually presents as headache, nausea, and vomiting secondary to raised

intracranial pressure (there may be papilledema); seizures, visual disturbances, and ataxia also occur. Cranial nerve palsies occur and commonly involve the oculomotor (III), abducens (VI), and facial (VII) nerves.   Diagnosis is made by LP: check for leukemic cells, elevated protein, decreased sugar, and an elevated pressure. Treatment with intrathecal methotrexate and radiotherapy is usually effective, and may be given prophylactically to leukemic patients in hematologic remission, before CNS complications occur.

Note: The hypothalamic-pituitary axis may be involved, giving hyperphagia (weight gain) or diabetes insipidus. In addition, there may be infiltration surrounding cord and roots; look for signs and symptoms of cord compression and/or root dysfunction.

3.   Infection. These patients are prone to CNS infection -- bacterial, fungal (cryptococcus), and listerial.   Whenever CNS symptoms are present, even if only drowsiness and headache, perform an LP to look for meningeal leukemia or infection.

Note: Herpes zoster is common, at times affecting roots with prior leukemic infiltration.

Lymphoma

Patients with lymphoma are subject to the same complications as those with leukemia except for intracerebral hemorrhage.

Spinal cord compression by lymphoma is especially common, as are compressive syndromes in other parts of the nervous system: brachial plexus, recurrent laryngeal nerve (vocal cord paralysis), phrenic nerve, cervical sympathetics (Horner's syndrome), and lumbosacral roots. Treatment of choice is radiation.   The compressive syndromes are more common in lymphomas than in leukemias.

Although intracerebral lymphoma is rare, it has been reported with reticulum cell sarcoma (histiocytic lymphoma).

Note: Meningeal involvement by tumors other than lymphoma and leukemia (carcinomatous meningitis) occurs. As with meningeal leukemia (see above), look for symptoms of raised intracranial pressure, multiple cranial nerve palsies, radiculopathy, and cerebrospinal fluid abnormalities (malignant cells and high protein). Treatment consists of intrathecal methotrexate and radiotherapy.

NON-METASTATIC COMPLICATIONS
OF MALIGNANCY

"Remote" Effects. This unique group of symptoms reflect the remote effects of malignancy on the nervous system. The etiology of these distant effects varies and

// Neurologic syndromes
may be the first manifestation of a malignancy
elsewhere //

may be related to immunologic, hormonal, or toxic factors elaborated by the tumor. It is known, however, that these neurologic syndromes may be the first manifestation of a malignancy elsewhere (e.g., peripheral neuropathy associated with lung tumor) and sometimes disappear when the primary tumor is removed. Certain neoplasms are more commonly associated with neurologic findings. However, as more syndromes are being reported, a wider spectrum of "etiologic malignancies" is becoming apparent.

Cerebellar Degeneration

Clinically, there is unsteadiness in gait and difficulty using limbs, progressing to slurring of speech and trouble in eating. Nystagmus may not be present. Cerebellar degeneration has been reported with tumors of lung, ovary, breast, colon, and with lymphoma. Although the cerebellar dysfunction is most striking, there may be other evidence of associated CNS dysfunction, including mental changes, muscle weakness, and extensor plantar responses.

Myasthenic (Eaton-Lambert)
Syndrome

This syndrome is most frequently associated with lung tumor in men. It presents as generalized weakness and easy fatigability, the weakness being most prominent proximally. Trouble with eye movements or difficulty swallowing is less common. The characteristic feature of this syndrome is that a few muscle contractions must be

carried out before full strength is reached, after which
the patient fatigues (in myasthenia gravis, full strength
is present at the outset and diminishes with exercise).
This can be demonstrated by electrodiagnostic studies.
Treatment with calcium and guanidine is more beneficial
than anticholinesterase medication. The myasthenic
syndrome may occur in the absence of malignancy and recent
evidence suggests an autoimmune basis for this syndrome.

Sensory Neuropathy

There is numbness and tingling of the upper and lower
extremities associated with a sensory ataxia; reflexes are
absent and there may be proximal muscle wasting in the
lower extremities. A sensorimotor neuropathy has also
been associated with malignancy.

Dementia

Dementia may be associated with malignancy (carcinoma
of the lung), often secondary to "limbic encephalitis"
which gives severely impaired memory. There may be
associated diffuse changes in the nervous system, and a
concomitant sensory neuropathy.

Polymyositis and Dermatomyositis

Both of these conditions are associated with neoplasm
and may antedate the appearance of the tumor. Myositis
presents as proximal muscle weakness. The muscles are not
usually tender, only weak. If tumor eradication is not
possible or does not help, steroids may be of benefit.

Remember, the importance of these remote effects of
malignancy is the clue they offer that a malignancy is
present, even though they may appear when the tumor is
well established. A characteristic feature of these
syndromes is that they are seldom "pure" -- they spill
over to involve more than one area of the nervous system.

Metabolic encephalopathy. Patients with cancer are
prone to develop lethargy, confusion, and behavior
disturbances as the result of metabolic abnormalities
related to, but not directly resulting from the underlying
cancer. Examples include uremia, hepatic and respiratory
failure; electrolyte disturbances such as hypercalcemia,
hyponatremia, hypoglycemia; drug overdoses. Also, as
discussed under the section on leukemia, patients with

cancer are prone to develop infections of various types, and sepsis may cause a metabolic encephalopathy. Metabolic brain disease is suggested by clouding of consciousness, a fluctuating picture, myoclonus, a lack of focal signs, and confirmatory laboratory studies, such as a normal CAT scan and an abnormal EEG which shows bilateral slowing without focal features.

Vascular Disorders. Cancer patients are prone to develop vascular disorders such as cerebral infarction secondary to disseminated intravascular coagulation, venous sinus thromboses or emboli from non-bacterial endocarditis. They are also prone to intracerebral, subarachnoid or subdural hemorrhage, as discussed previously under leukemia.

Other. Cancer patients may develop side effects of therapy, such as radiation myelopathy, neuropathy, and encephalopathy, and peripheral neuropathy secondary to chemotherapeutic agents (esp. vincristine and cis-platinum).

Note: Progressive multifocal leukoencephalopathy (PML) is usually seen in patients with a compromised immune system. This occurs in patients with malignancies such as lymphomas or secondary to immunosuppression from chemotherapy. Clinically, patients develop multifocal white matter lesions over a period of 6 months to 2 years and the clinical picture may be confused with multiple strokes.

REFERENCES

1. Cairncross JG, Kim JH, Posner JB: Radiation therapy for brain metastasis. Ann Neurol 7:529, 1980.
2. Pochedly C: Leukemia and Lymphoma in the Nervous System, Springfield, Charles Thomas, 1977.
3. Posner JB: Neurologic complications of systemic cancer. Disease-a-Month. Yearbook Medical Publishers 25(2) Nov. 1978.
4. Posner JB, Shapiro WR: Brain tumor: Current status of treatment and its complications. Arch Neurol 32:781, 1975.
5. Symposium on cancer and the nervous system. Brain 88, 1965.
6. Wilson CB: Brain tumors. N Engl J Med 300:1469, 1979.

Chapter 22

Neurology of Uremia

MENTAL STATUS CHANGES

One of the most common features of renal failure is an altered mental status. It may range from irritability and difficulty in concentration (e.g., performing serial sevens) to actual psychotic reactions. Mental status changes in uremics fluctuate; periods of confusion are interspersed with periods of lucidity.

<u>Acute changes in mental status</u> are generally encountered postdiuresis or postdialysis when there have been rapid electrolyte shifts, even though actual electrolyte values are improved ("dysequilibrium syndrome"). Metabolically, brain shifts of urea and/or pH lag or often do not parallel systemic changes. Slowly developing renal failure causes fewer mental status changes than does rapidly developing failure.

<u>EEG changes</u> are usual with an altered mental status and usually parallel the degree of metabolic encephalopathy. Most patients with a BUN greater than 60 mg/100 ml have EEG abnormalities (generalized slowing).

Although the majority of mental status changes (increased irritability and lack of ability to concentrate in the "stable uremic", or periods of marked disorientation secondary to rapid metabolic shifts) are not secondary to treatable nervous system disease, keep other possibilities in mind:

1. <u>Infection</u>. Fungal or other uncommon CNS pathogens are not uncommon in uremics. Perform an LP when

there is unexplained confusion or fever in the uremic
patient after performing a CAT scan to rule out
subdural hematoma. Remember to do an India ink
preparation for cryptococcus or test for cryptococcal
antigen if there are cells in the CSF (see Chapter
26).

2.   Subdural hematoma. Uremics have an increased
bleeding tendency, and subdural collections may
develop with mild head trauma or during dialysis.
If a subdural hematoma is suspected because of
lateralizing signs or persistent lethargy with
headache, obtain a brain or CAT scan.

CONVULSIONS

Convulsions are a common feature of renal disease;
they signify different processes, depending on the type
(generalized or focal) and the clinical setting (e.g.,
postdialysis). Patients with acute anuria may develop
convulsions on the eighth to eleventh day of renal
failure, or with the onset of diuresis and subsequent
rapid electrolyte shifts. These convulsions tend to be
generalized.

Convulsions also appear late in the course of
chronic renal disease and frequently are associated
with abnormal blood chemistries: acidosis, hypokalemia,
hyponatremia. No one abnormal electrolyte is consistently
associated with seizures, but the greater the
potassium/calcium ratio the greater is the risk of
convulsion.

Seizures are common postdialysis.

In patients with either acute or chronic renal
failure, the first convulsion may be a preterminal
event.

Treatment of Convulsions

1.   The drug of choice is phenytoin, which is
metabolized by the liver, not kidney, and is not
removed during dialysis. Administer 1000 mg (15
mg/kg) I.V. over 30 to 45 minutes if immediate
therapeutic levels are needed, then 300-400 mg daily.

Follow the phenytoin levels (see Chapter 11).

2. Generalized or multifocal seizures (one side, then
    the other) occurring during a time of metabolic flux
    (dialysis, diuresis) are generally self-limited.
    Treat with phenytoin, and when the patient has
    stabilized anticonvulsants may be withdrawn.

3. Persistently focal seizures should be worked up:
    LP, EEG, and CAT scan or brain scan. Further
    investigation (arteriography) may be needed if there
    are focal neurologic signs. Patients may have tiny
    areas of cortical hemorrhage that account for the
    focal seizure.

4. Check for predisposing electrolyte disturbances and
    correct where appropriate.

5. Some physicians give phenytoin prophylactically to
    patients who are about to experience rapid
    electrolyte shifts (e.g., during dialysis).

PERIPHERAL NEUROPATHY

Early. Patients often begin with a "restless leg
syndrome". The leg feels uncomfortable when the patient
is still and relief occurs after ambulation. Another
early neuropathic syndrome consists of painful, burning
paresthesias of the feet similar to that seen in
alcoholics and associated with dietary insufficiency.
Resolution may follow proper diet and vitamin supplements.

Late. A more severe peripheral neuropathy develops
over weeks to months and is not diet-dependent. Check for
distal loss of all sensory modalities (pinprick, position,
vibration). Legs are affected significantly more than the
arms. It is a motor as well as sensory neuropathy and may
lead to actual paraplegia (at this stage the arms may also
become involved). Treatment is extremely difficult and
although dialysis helps some, it is generally ineffective;
transplantation reverses the neuropathy. Nerve conduction
velocities are slow in most uremics, regardless of whether
they have symptomatic neuropathy.

OTHER NEUROLOGIC FEATURES
OF UREMIA

Dialysis may precipitate convulsions or a toxic

encephalopathy. In this "reverse urea syndrome" urea
leaves the brain more slowly than it leaves the blood;
fluid is thus drawn into brain, resulting in acute
swelling. There may also be a lag in pH equilibrium. The
encephalopathy usually clears in 24 to 48 hours.
Remember, subdural hematoma sometimes follows dialysis.

Asterixis frequently accompanies uremic
encephalopathy as do muscle fasciculations and myoclonus.

Muscle cramps may occur and generally are not
related to a specific electrolyte abnormality, although
they are more frequent when water intoxication is present.
Chvostek's sign may be positive in uremia, and correlates
with the acidosis and elevated potassium/calcium ratio
rather than with decreased calcium alone. There may be
mild proximal muscle weakness.

"Uremic amaurosis" has been reported with the acute
development of blindness; this may be related to focal
cerebral edema. Complete recovery usually occurs.

Cerebral emboli may occur during the declotting of
shunts used for hemodialysis.

Dialysis dementia has been reported in patients
with uremia and represents a progressive neurologic
deterioration in patients on hemodialysis. It consists of
dementia, myoclonus, speech disorders, neuropsychiatric
abnormalities, gait abnormalities, and EEG changes.
Etiology is unknown; some cases may be due to metal
intoxication, but in most cases the etiology is obscure.
Clinical and EEG improvement may follow treatment with
diazepam or other anticonvulsants.

Carpal tunnel syndrome is more common in patients
on hemodialysis.

REFERENCES

1.   Bolton CF: Peripheral neuropathies associated with
      chronic renal failure. Canad J Neurol Sci 7:89,
      1980.
2.   Dewberry FL, et al.: The dialysis dementia syndrome:
      report of fourteen cases and review of the
      literature. J Am Soc Artif Int Organs 3:102, 1980.

3. Lazaro RP, Kirshner HS: Proximal muscle weakness in
    uremia. Case reports and review of the literature.
    Arch Neurol 37:555, 1980.
4. Noriega-Sanchez A, Martinez-Maldonado M, Haffe RM:
    Clinical and electroencephalographic changes in
    progressive uremic encephalopathy. Neurology
    28:667, 1978.
5. Raskin NH, Fishman RA: Neurologic disorders in renal
    failure. N Engl J Med 294:143, 204, 1976.

Chapter 23

Neurology of Alcoholism

SEIZURES

Seizures are common in the alcoholic and represent at least two different phenomena. It is important to distinguish the two types of "alcoholic seizures" because treatment and work-up are different.

"Rum Fits"

Rum fits are brief, self-limited, generalized seizures secondary to abstinence from alcohol or a reduction in the usual intake. They do not represent a true convulsive disorder, and most occur 12 to 48 hours after decreased alcohol intake, although they can occur earlier or later (rarely after 96 hours). A night's sleep without alcohol may be enough to precipitate a seizure. Remember, rum fits can occur in the "businessman-drinker" who comes to the hospital for another reason. Alcohol withdrawal seizures tend to appear in groups of two or three and then stop. The patient is usually tremulous and jittery. The interictal EEG in these patients is normal, and if the history is characteristic, the patient requires no work-up or anticonvulsant medication. Often a patient is placed on anticonvulsants in the hospital after the first seizure, but when it becomes apparent that he had a "withdrawal seizure", anticonvulsants are tapered and discontinued. Patients with "rum fits" are markedly sensitive to photic stimulation during EEG. Patients with "rum fits" are at a higher risk for developing delirium tremens.

Seizures Precipitated by Alcohol

These alcohol-induced seizures are usually focal and reflect an intrinsic CNS lesion. Seizures of this type may occur during the period of intoxication. Such patients generally have an abnormal EEG, require a basic neurologic work-up for seizure, and treatment with anticonvulsants. Focal seizures in the alcoholic often represent post-traumatic epilepsy due to multiple falls. It is important to remember that focal seizures represent CNS pathology, and alcoholics are especially prone to subdural hematoma and meningitis. Persistently focal seizures in an alcoholic should be considered to be caused by a subdural until proven otherwise. Alcoholics have the same risk for brain tumor as does the general population.

// Was the seizure focal
or generalized? When
did it occur? //

Remember the questions to answer when treating the seizure of an alcoholic: Was the seizure focal or generalized? When did it occur in relation to drinking?

ALCOHOLIC TREMULOUSNESS
-- DELIRIUM TREMENS

The spectrum of alcohol withdrawal symptoms include mild tremulousness to fatal delirium tremens (DTs). The underlying physiology in these states is related to abstinence from alcohol, not to specific dietary or vitamin insufficiency. Similar withdrawal states can occur after stopping other CNS depressants (e.g., barbiturates, diazepam). DTs and withdrawal seizures can be produced in normal individuals on good diets who are placed on large amounts of alcohol and then withdrawn. Seizures are a point on the spectrum of withdrawal symptomatology. When an alcoholic stops drinking, he is subject to the following:

1. Tremulousness is one of the first signs of alcohol withdrawal, beginning approximately eight hours after cessation of drinking (often after a night's sleep), and reaching its peak at 24 hours. The patient is

jittery, startles easily, and often shows a gross irregular tremor of the hands. Although these symptoms are most severe at 24 hours, it may take seven to ten days before the patient is back to normal. Drinkers who suffer from tremulousness upon arising in the morning may take a drink to "calm their nerves".

2.   Seizures have already been discussed.

3.   Hallucinations appear during the withdrawal period and are commonly visual, although they may be auditory. Sometimes the patient hallucinates in the presence of an otherwise clear sensorium.

4.   Delirium tremens completes the spectrum. This reaction occurs about 72 to 96 hours after cessation of drinking. Those who have had a chronic period of drinking before cessation experience the most severe form of DTs. They suffer from tremulousness, hallucinations, and marked autonomic hyperactivity (tachycardia, hyperhidrosis, fever, dilated pupils). DTs are a relatively uncommon sequelae of alcoholic withdrawal, but can be fatal; they are often preceded by an alcoholic withdrawal seizure.

Treatment of DTs

Treatment consists of supportive care. Adequate diet and vitamins have no effect on the course of alcohol withdrawal, but must be given to prevent other complications. Pay careful attention to fluid and electrolyte balance, and search thoroughly for underlying disease (e.g., subdural hematoma, pneumonia, and meningitis). These diseases are not uncommon and often are the factors that make DTs fatal. We use chlordiazepoxide (Librium), 50 mg PO or IM q four to six hours, or paraldehyde, 10 cc PO or PR q four to six hours, to lessen the agitation (watch for oversedation). There is no evidence that steroids are of benefit. It may not be possible to prevent DTs, but one can lessen the severity of agitation with medication; by controlling fluid and electrolyte balance the chances for recovery are good.

VITAMIN DEFICIENCY
SYNDROMES AND ALCOHOLISM

In addition to the alcohol withdrawal syndrome, there is a group of vitamin-dependent syndromes seen almost exclusively in alcoholics in this country. (They also appear in nonalcoholics with poor diets.)

Wernicke's Encephalopathy

This thiamine deficiency syndrome consists of a characteristic clinical triad:

1. <u>Ocular changes</u>. Look for nystagmus on horizontal and/or vertical gaze, sixth nerve palsies that are generally bilateral and paralysis of conjugate gaze. In severe forms there may be total ophthalmoplegia.

2. <u>Gait difficulties</u>. Check for ataxia: a wide-based gait, falling, or inability to walk or stand.

3. <u>Mental symptoms</u>. Patients usually manifest a quiet confusional state. <u>Korsakoff's psychosis</u> is an extension of the mental symptoms of Wernicke's disease and becomes apparent later if the Wernicke's syndrome is untreated. The main feature is a marked disorder of memory and confabulation. The patient is unable to learn new material such as the doctor's name or who visited ten minutes earlier. CAT scans in chronic alcoholics often show evidence of cerebral and cerebellar atrophy.

In addition to the above triad, thiamine deficiency can produce dysautonomias, including cardiac failure and EKG changes.

<u>Treatment</u> consists of thiamine (50 mg IV and 50 mg IM) to improve the oculomotor dysfunction -- it may resolve within minutes to hours (a diagnostic as well as therapeutic maneuver) -- and to prevent the development of Korsakoff's psychosis. The 50 mg IM dose should be repeated daily until the patient resumes a normal diet. Occasionally, larger doses may be needed initially to improve oculomotor dysfunction. Be careful when giving intravenous fluids to alcoholics; glucose may cause depletion of

// In alcoholics: add
thiamine to intravenous
solutions //

thiamine stores and precipitate Wernicke's syndrome
(add thiamine to the intravenous solution).
Furthermore, Wernicke's syndrome can occur in
non-alcoholics who are dependent on parental
alimentation for several days (e.g., surgical or burn
unit patients).

Polyneuropathy

Polyneuropathy occurs in alcoholics secondary to
nutritional factors and may also be related in part to the
toxic effects of alcohol. Most patients are asymptomatic
but lose ankle and sometimes knee jerks. When symptoms
occur, they consist of burning feet, pain, paresthesias,
and mild distal weakness. The feet may be so sensitive
that bed covers touching the feet are painful. In severe
cases the weakness may progress to wrist-drop and
foot-drop. Polyneuropathy and Wernicke's syndrome often
occur in the same patient.

Treatment consists of improving the diet, complete
abstinence from alcohol, and adding vitamin supplements.
Some clinicians give phenytoin during the acute stage;
recovery is slow but usually occurs with abstinence and
proper diet.

OTHER NEUROLOGIC COMPLICATIONS
OF ALCOHOLISM

Cerebellar degeneration affects men more frequently
than women. There is a wide-based gait with truncal
instability and a less prominent limb ataxia. The
symptoms appear over weeks to months, although they may
come on acutely. The acutely occurring syndrome has a
better prognosis and may not represent actual cerebellar
structural damage, as does the chronic form. Treatment
consists of dietary and vitamin support. Further
abstinence from alcohol is crucial.

Some patients may have slowly developing myopathy with
proximal muscle weakness, often in conjunction with

alcoholic cardiac myopathy.   There is an acute form with muscle pain, weakness, and elevated CPK.   Treatment is symptomatic.

Rare complications of alcoholism or malnutrition include central pontine myelinolysis and the Marchiafava-Bignami corpus callosum syndrome.

REFERENCES

1.   Behse F, Buchthal F: Alcoholic neuropathy: Clinical, electrophysiological, and biopsy findings. Ann Neurol 2:95, 1977.
2.   Carlen PL, Wortzman G, Holgate RC: Reversible cerebral atrophy in recently abstinent alcoholics measured by CT scan.   Science 200:1076, 1978.
3.   Thomas DW, Friedman DX: Treatment of the alcohol withdrawal syndrome. JAMA 188:316, 1964.
4.   Victor M, Adams RD: The effect of alcohol upon the nervous system. Res Publ Assoc Res Nerv Ment Dis 32:526, 1953.
5.   Victor M, Adams R, Collins G: The Wernicke-Korsakoff Syndrome. Philadelphia, F.A. Davis Company, 1971.

Chapter 24

Raised Intracranial Pressure

Raised intracranial pressure may be secondary to focal mass lesions or more diffuse processes. Signs and symptoms include headache, nausea and vomiting, lethargy, diplopia (usually secondary to a sixth nerve palsy) and papilledema. As intracranial pressure continues to rise there may be bradycardia (50-60 beats/minute), elevation of blood pressure, increase in systolic pressure associated with lowering or slight elevation of diastolic pressure, and a slowing of the respiratory rate. This is termed the Cushing reflex, but cannot be depended upon for the diagnosis of raised intracranial pressure.

AGENTS USED IN TREATING INTRACRANIAL PRESSURE

Hyperventilation

Hyperventilation may be used in acute situations (e.g., head trauma) and is often employed during neurosurgical procedures. By lowering the P_{CO2} to 25 to 30 mm Hg, there is reduced cerebral blood flow, an immediate reduction in intracerebral blood volume and thus a decrease of intracranial pressure. Lowering P_{CO2} below 25 mm Hg may be harmful as it reduces cerebral blood flow. If a patient brought to the emergency ward has rapid neurologic deterioration from increased intracranial

pressure, whether due to trauma or to other intracranial
processes, intubation and hyperventilation is often an
effective means of lowering the pressure until such agents
as mannitol take effect and specific neurosurgical
treatment is instituted.

Mannitol

Mannitol, an osmotic dehydrating agent, is given
1-2 gm per kg IV over five to ten minutes, then 50-300
mg/kg IV every six hours, depending on serum osmolarity.
Onset of action is 15-30 minutes. It draws intracerebral
water into the intravascular space because of its
hypertonicity and for the same reason induces diuresis.
It is usually not given for more than 24 to 48 hours and
is used in acute situations to "buy time" (e.g., after
head trauma, deterioration from an expanding intracranial
process), often prior to neurosurgical intervention.
Urea is similar to mannitol in its use, mode of action,
and dose. These agents must be given with caution to
patients with renal and cardiac disease. There may be
"rebound" after their use (viz., return of water
intracerebrally) because small amounts cross the blood
brain barrier.

Steroids

Steroids (dexamethasone) are used both acutely and
chronically (10 mg IV as initial dose, then 4 mg IV, IM or
orally every six hours). The onset of action is about 12
hours. Dexamethasone is given in acute situations and may
become the mainstay of treatment after 12 to 24 hours. It
is used palliatively to treat brain tumor, after
neurosurgical procedures, and often concomitantly with
radiation therapy to the brain. The mechanism of steroid
action in these situations is poorly understood. All
patients receiving steroids for more than a few hours
should receive cimetidine and oral antacids. Steroids are
probably not beneficial in treating adults with trauma
induced cerebral edema.

Glycerol

Glycerol, an osmotic dehydrating agent, is given
orally or via nasogastric tube in a dose of 1 gm per kg
every six hours. It is slower acting than mannitol/urea
(onset of action is approximately 12 hours), but has the

advantage that it can be used for longer periods and can be given orally. It does not have the side effects of prolonged steroid administration, and there is little "rebound". It is used to treat swelling associated with cerebrovascular accidents, after neurosurgical procedures, or concomitantly with steroids.

Ventricular Puncture

Ventricular puncture may be done by a neurosurgeon when acute hydrocephalus occurs and mechanical release of raised intracranial pressure is needed. Causes include posterior fossa mass lesions, meningitis, and subarachnoid hemorrhage. Ventricular puncture may be done in the emergency room or on the ward.

Barbiturates

A recent contribution to intracranial pressure (ICP) control is the use of barbiturates. They are usually used when other attempts to lower ICP have failed and should be used in conjunction with an intraventricular pressure monitor in an intensive care unit. Pentobarbital is the most widely used agent. Its mechanism of action in reducing ICP is unknown.

TREATMENT

When transtentorial herniation is in progress (see below), mannitol should be given immediately and neurosurgical consultation obtained. This refers to trauma, abrupt changes intracerebrally secondary to a vascular event, or deterioration after lumbar puncture. Concomitant with mannitol administration, dexamethasone should be given. If clinically appropriate, intubation and hyperventilation are also indicated.

In the stroke patient with a component of cerebral swelling or intracerebral hemorrhage (demonstrated by midline shift on CAT scan accompanying a decreased level of consciousness) some physicians use corticosteroids or glycerol during the acute period. Cerebral swelling secondary to thrombosis or embolus is most pronounced approximately 48 hours after the event; intracerebral hemorrhage may raise the intracranial pressure acutely.

Patients with **brain tumors** (primary or secondary) are often treated with steroids after diagnosis, during radiation therapy, and sometimes on a chronic basis. Interestingly, metastatic brain tumor tends to respond better to steroids than does primary brain tumor.

Continuous monitoring of increased intracranial pressure with pressure monitoring devices is now possible and may be very useful in certain patients with severe head injury. Either an intraventricular cannula or a subarachnoid bolt can be used to monitor pressure and aid in therapeutic decisions.

HERNIATION SYNDROMES

There are three clinical syndromes of transtentorial herniation. Two represent loss of neurologic function which begins in the cerebral hemispheres and progresses to involve upper, then lower brain stem with death the usual result. The third consists of upward herniation of posterior fossa structures and can also be fatal.

A.   Uncal (lateral) syndrome of herniation

1.   A unilaterally dilated pupil is the first sign secondary to a mass in the middle fossa pushing against the uncus and trapping the third nerve. A contralateral hemiplegia is usually present. Respiration and consciousness are unimpaired.

2.   Progressive pressure leads to increasing stupor, a more complete third nerve palsy and sometimes an ipsilateral hemiplegia with bilateral Babinski responses. The ipsilateral hemiplegia is secondary to tentorial pressure against the opposite cerebral peduncle (Kernohan's notch). Respiration may be normal or of the central neurogenic hyperventilation pattern. There is often decerebrate posturing (arms extended at the side with inward turning, either spontaneously or when a noxious stimulus is applied). Decorticate posturing (arms flexed at the elbow "pointing" to the cortex) is not usually seen with the uncal syndrome.

3.   Further pressure leads to prominent brainstem dysfunction with dilatation of both pupils, loss

of brain stem reflexes (e.g., absent doll's eyes, no response to ice-water calorics), ataxic respiratory patterns, and bilateral decerebrate rigidity. Treatment at this stage is rarely of benefit.

B.   Central syndrome of herniation

1.   Pressure is exerted centrally on the diencephalon, rather than laterally as occurs in the uncal syndrome. The first sign is a change in alertness or behavior. Respiration is usually normal and contains frequent sighs or yawns. There may be Cheyne-Stokes respirations. Brainstem function is intact, although pupils are small but reactive to light and there may be roving eye movements. There usually is bilateral hyperreflexia and Babinski responses and rigidity of the extremities. With progression there is decorticate posturing.

2.   Involvement of upper brain stem leads to dilatation of both pupils and impairment of oculocephalic and oculovestibular reflexes (i.e., absent or abnormal doll's eyes or caloric response). Central neurogenic hyperventilation often occurs and decorticate posturing progresses to decerebrate posturing. There may be wide fluctuations in body temperature.

3.   Further progression leads to loss of all brain stem function with ataxic breathing, then apnea and death.

C.   Posterior fossa herniation syndrome

1.   Posterior fossa lesions may cause damage both by direct compression of the brainstem and by upward herniation through the tentorial hiatus. Upward herniation from the posterior fossa obliterates the ambient cisterns and aquaduct causing hydrocephalus with obtundation and/or coma.

2.   Midbrain compression produces an upward gaze deficit, while involvement of pontine pathways may cause six nerve palsies, ocular bobbing and

other oculomotor signs. In addition, there may be anisocoria leading to midposition and fixed pupils.

These syndromes can develop over hours or minutes, depending on the pathologic process. The uncal syndrome is typically seen secondary to space occupying lesions, such as intracranial hemorrhage or subdural hematoma, while central herniation is seen with diffuse increased intracranial pressure, e.g., Reye's syndrome or acute hydrocephalus. The posterior syndrome occurs with posterior fossa mass lesions.

REFERENCES

1. Mauss NK, Mitchell PH: Increased intracranial pressure: an update. Heart Lung 5:919, 1976.
2. Saper JR, Yosselson S: Raised intracranial pressure, diagnosis and management. Postgrad Med 57:89, April, 1975.
3. Tourtellotte WW, Reinglass JL, Newkirk TA: Cerebral dehydration action of glycerol. Clin Pharmacol Ther 13:159, 1972.
4. Wise BL, Chater N: The value of hypertonic mannitol solution in decreasing brain mass and lowering cerebrospinal fluid pressure. J Neurosurg 19:1038, 1962.

Chapter 25

Head Trauma

Head injury is a dynamic process. The most important parameters to monitor are the patient's level of consciousness and mental status. Below are important guidelines in dealing with the patient with head trauma:

1. In <u>severe head trauma</u>, control of airway and IV placement are first priorities. One should assume the patient has a fractured cervical spine and avoid turning the head; obtain cervical spine films in addition to skulls. Search for accompanying traumatic injury to abdominal and thoracic organs. If a patient has head injury and shock, assume they are unrelated.

2. In all cases of head trauma <u>neurologic examination</u> should be performed and must include (a) careful documentation of the patient's level of consciousness and ability to carry out mental tasks; (b) a careful look
                    // Carefully evaluate
                    mental status //

    at the tympanic membranes for evidence of basilar skull fracture (blood or CSF); (c) scalp examination for evidence of localized areas of trauma; (d) precise recording of pupillary size and reaction; (e) check for hemiparesis and presence or absence of upgoing toes.

3. <u>Concussion</u> is defined as an immediate and transient loss of consciousness or other neurologic function following head injury. There may be amnesia for events that occurred prior to and after the head injury.

4. <u>Observation in the hospital</u> for a period of 24 to 48 hours and <u>neurosurgical consultation</u> is appropriate for a patient with any focal abnormalities on neurologic examination, a period of unconsciousness, an abnormal mental status, skull fracture, or head trauma that is felt significant despite a normal examination. The decision to hospitalize or send home a patient who has not been unconscious and who has a normal neurologic exam must be made after careful consideration of the severity of the trauma and of who will look after and monitor the patient at home.

5. One of the most feared complications of head injury is the development of an acute <u>subdural</u> or <u>epidural hematoma</u>, which then may cause herniation (see Chapter 24) and fatal brainstem compression. Clinically, this process manifests itself as headache, decreased level of consciousness, and, late in the course, a dilated pupil that is usually on the side of the hematoma secondary to pressure on the third nerve. <u>Epidural hematoma</u> most commonly represents arterial bleeding secondary to tearing the middle meningeal artery on the undersurface of the temporal bone. The patient may steadily deteriorate following the trauma or experience a "lucid interval" only to deteriorate later. Most (although not all) patients will have a fracture over the groove of the middle meningeal artery. <u>Subdural hematoma</u> is secondary to venous or arterial bleeding and similarly has the potential for brainstem compression. Subdural and epidural hematomas are diagnosed by CAT scan and, in certain instances, by arteriography.

6. There is potential danger and no value in doing a lumbar puncture in the patient with acute head trauma.

7.   Skull films are an important part of the evaluation
      of a patient with significant head trauma and may
      show such abnormalities as: depressed fractures,
      linear fractures in the middle fossa or base of the
      skull, air fluid level in the ethmoid sinus. Skull
      films should not, however, be requested before a CAT
      scan in a patient with severe injury and should not
      necessarily be done in all patients with minor
      injuries.

REFERENCES

1.   Bruce DA, et al.: Resuscitation from coma due to
      head injury. Crit Care Med 6:254, 1978.
2.   Dublin AB, French, BN, Rennick JM: Computed
      tomography in head trauma. Radiology 122:365,
      1977.
3.   Jennet B: Assessment of the severity of head injury.
      J Neurol Neurosurg Psychiat 39:647, 1976.
4.   McLaurin RL, ed: Head Injuries, New York, Grune and
      Stratton, 1976.
5.   Tindall GT, Patton JM, Dunion JJ, et al.: Monitoring
      patients with head injuries. Clin Neurosurg
      22:332, 1975.

Chapter 26

Lumbar Puncture

INDICATIONS

1. When CNS infection is suspected one must examine the CSF. Exception: If one suspects brain abscess or other significant mass lesion (see p. 144).

2. An LP is performed to determine if CNS bleeding has occurred -- e.g., to diagnose subarachnoid hemorrhage or to rule out bleeding prior to anticoagulation.

3. An LP is done when CSF chemistries have diagnostic value -- e.g., gamma globulin in multiple sclerosis.

4. Lumbar puncture is needed for the study of CSF dynamics -- e.g., when checking for spinal block (performance of Quekenstedt test) or normal pressure hydrocephalus (performance of Katzman infusion or radionucleotide cisternography).

5. Therapeutically, an LP may be done to inject methotrexate for CNS leukemia or amphotericin B for fungal meningitis; to remove fluid as treatment for benign raised intracranial pressure or for the headache of subarachnoid hemorrhage.

CONTRAINDICATIONS

1. Infection at the site of the lumbar puncture.

2. Severe thrombocytopenia or uncorrected bleeding disorder.

3.   When a cerebral <u>mass lesion</u> is suspected,
     particularly in a patient with lateralized
     neurologic signs.

     . <u>Brain abscesses</u> (usually seen in congenital
        heart disease with right to left shunts, otitis
        media, or lung disease) may produce
        transtentorial or foramen magnum herniation
        after LP.

     . <u>Brain tumors</u> may lead to herniation after LP,
        especially when located in the posterior fossa.

     . <u>Subdural hematoma</u> is not usually diagnosed by
        LP and the removal of fluid may be harmful.

     . <u>Intracranial hemorrhage</u> is best diagnosed by
        CAT scan.

     In these instances, a CAT scan or, if not
available, definition of the midline via skull film and
a search for a mass lesion via EEG and brain scan should
be done before the LP.

4.   Lumbar puncture must not be done in the presence of
     <u>papilledema</u> (a check of the fundi must precede
     each LP). An LP may ultimately be done in a
     patient with papilledema (e.g., in pseudotumor or
     if CSF examination is crucial), but only after
     neurologic and/or neurosurgical consultation.

COMPLICATIONS

     <u>Post-LP headache</u> occurs in 10% to 30% of
patients. It is characteristically exacerbated by
sitting or standing, and relieved by lying flat. It is
seen within the first one to three days after the LP; it
usually lasts two to five days, although it may persist
for weeks. Treatment consists of bed rest and fluids.
(The mechanism of the headache is believed to be
continued CSF leakage through the dural hole at the site
of the LP, with subsequent intracranial traction on the
meninges.) Post-LP headache may be minimized by using a
small gauge needle (22 or 20), inserting the needle
parallel to the dural fibers so they are spread apart
rather than torn, having the patient turn prone before
removing the needle and removing less than 10 cc of
fluid. Having the patient lie in bed post-LP may or may

not be useful. Patients with migraine are particularly prone to post-LP headaches.

When there is an unexpected <u>raised pressure</u> (it must stay elevated after the patient has relaxed with legs extended, and ten minutes have elapsed from the onset of the LP), remove minimal fluid needed for studies. Neurologic and/or neurosurgical consultation should be obtained, the use of mannitol and/or steroids considered, and the patient watched carefully over the ensuing hours for signs of deterioration. Patients with meningitis may have markedly elevated pressures, but these pressures are not as dangerous as raised intracranial pressure secondary to a focal lesion. Remember, hypercarbia, water intoxication, and hypertensive encephalopathy are remediable causes of raised intracranial pressure. When the intracranial pressure is raised and there is neurologic deterioration immediately or during the hours after the LP, treatment with osmotic dehydrating agents and steroids is indicated (see Chapter 24).

If the patient has a partial or almost complete <u>spinal block</u> secondary to compression of the cord (e.g., by tumor) CSF removal may cause rapid worsening of the block. Signs of block include abnormal manometric findings and xanthochromic fluid under low pressure (see Chapter 13 for treatment).

METHOD OF LUMBAR PUNCTURE

1. The puncture is carried out in the midline between the L3-L4 or L4-L5 interspaces located by the level of the iliac crest.

2. Insert the level of the needle parallel to the long axis of the spine.

3. If manometric studies and myelography are not being performed, use a 20- or 22- gauge needle.

4. Note the opening and closing pressure as well as the amount of fluid removed.

5. Coughing or abdominal pressure cause delayed venous return around the cord and should increase CSF flow and pressure. These maneuvers show that the needle is in place, but they do not test for spinal

subarachnoid block. To do this, raise the jugular
pressure (via hand pressure or a blood pressure
cuff around the neck) and measure the rise and fall
of CSf pressure. Manometric studies are not done
routinely, and never if the baseline pressure is
elevated or when an intracranial lesion is
suspected.

6.   Proper positioning of the patient is crucial for
     successful lumbar puncture. The patient should be
     placed in the fetal position with his back at right
     angles to the bed. Insert the needle under the
     skin (after local anesthesia) and then decide on
     the angle of entry. Make sure the needle is
     strictly parallel to the bed and angled toward the
     patient's umbilicus. Once the needle has been
     advanced, if it does not enter the subarachnoid
     space or encounters bone, the direction of the
     needle cannot be changed. Pull the needle back to
     just beneath the skin and redirect it. With
     experience, one will learn to recognize the
     familiar "pop" as the needle enters the
     subarachnoid space. If the LP is not possible in
     the fetal position, have the patient sit up and
     lean forward grasping a pillow; try again in the
     sitting position (it is easier to gauge the
     midline). Remember, pressure measurements are
     difficult to interpret in the sitting position and
     it may be useful to have the patient lie down after
     the needle is inserted.

7.   When an LP is impossible because of bony anomalies
     or local infection, and CSF examination is crucial,
     one should arrange for a cisternal or cervical
     (C1-C2) tap under fluorscopy.

                    EXAMINATION OF THE CSF

                         The Fluid

1.   Collect three tubes: One tube is used for cell
     count, one for chemistries, and a third for
     bacteriologic studies. A fourth tube may be saved
     for future use, e.g., a sample may be lost, an
     unexpected chemistry value may require a repeat
     determination, or a new test may be wanted. If a
     traumatic tap is suspected, cells are counted in
     both the first and third tubes. In order to settle

the issue of a "traumatic tap", a repeat tap is done at a higher interspace, or sometimes a cisternal tap is performed.

2. If RBCs are present, count them in the first and third tubes. In subarachnoid or intracranial bleeding, the amount of blood remains constant in each tube, and the blood does not clot. Decreasing numbers of cells suggests a traumatic tap. After centrifugation, the CSF from a traumatic tap will be clear, while with true CNS bleeding the supernatant is xanthochromic if the bleeding occurred at least two to four hours previously. Finding crenated RBCs is of no distinguishing value, since they appear both with true bleeding and after traumatic taps.

3. Check to see if the CSF is clear by comparing it with water. A CSF protein level greater than 100 mg/100 ml usually causes the spinal fluid to look faintly yellow. Approximately 200 to 300 WBCs are needed to cause CSF cloudiness. Dark CSF may be seen with metastatic melanoma, jaundice with hyperbilirubinemia, and subdural hematoma may produce xanthochromia.

4. Always examine the CSF for cells within one hour after LP, and preferably sooner. Normally, there should be no polymorphonuclear neutrophils (PMNs) and no more than five mononuclear cells. It is very important to distinguish between RBCs and WBCs. After a total cell count is done, add acetic acid to the spinal fluid; this lyses the RBCs but leaves the WBCs intact. (Rinse a capillary tube with acetic acid and then draw the CSF into the tube.) Often one can distinguish between PMNs and lymphocytes by adding methylene blue to the fluid. When looking for tumor cells, or if the nature of the WBCs in the CSF is questioned, a Millipore, cytocentrifuge, or cytologic examination is indicated. When bacterial or tuberculous infection is suspected, perform a gram stain and an acid fast stain on the centrifuged sediment; when fungal disease is a possibility, do an India Ink preparation. (Place a coverslip over one drop of CSF on a slide. Place a drop of India ink next to the coverslip and allow it to seep under. Check at the interface for cryptococcus organisms.)

5.   When there are RBCs in the CSF and the patient has
      a normal CBC, expect approximately one WBC for
      every 700 RBCs (make further corrections for
      anemia). In addition, every 700 RBCs raises the
      protein by 1 mg/100 ml.

INTERPRETATION

Glucose

      Increased glucose levels are usually not
significant, merely reflecting systemic hyperglycemia.
With changing blood glucose, CSF glucose lags blood
glucose by approximately one hour and the level is
two-thirds that of blood glucose. In the face of systemic
hyperglycemia a concomitant blood glucose is needed to
demonstrate a relatively lowered CSF glucose that might
otherwise be considered normal.

      Decreased glucose levels are seen in bacterial
tuberculous, and fungal meningitis, and sometimes with
meningeal involvement by neoplasm or a nontuberculous
granulomatous process such as sarcoidosis. Although
characteristically normal in viral infections, the CSF
glucose has been reported low with certain CNS viral
infections (herpes, mumps, lymphocytic choriomeningitis).
Decreased CSF glucose is secondary to changes in
carbohydrate metabolism by neural tissue, WBC utilization
of glucose and alteration of glucose transport into the
CNS.

Protein

      Protein levels are increased in a wide variety of
neurologic diseases and usually reflect an abnormality in
the blood-brain barrier. Elevated levels are seen in
processes affecting nerve roots in peripheral neuropathy.
A survey of common processes producing increased CSF
protein follows. Normal CSF protein is less than 45
mg/100 ml.

1.   Diabetes frequently causes protein elevations (up
      to 150 mg/100 ml, although it may be even higher when
      significant peripheral neuropathy is present). Look
      for unrecognized diabetes when there is an unexpected
      protein elevation. The mechanism is probably related
      to dorsal root ganglia involvement.

2. **Brain tumor** frequently produces protein elevation
    of 100 to 200 mg/100 ml, although the level may be
    normal. Marked increases are seen in meningiomas,
    acoustic neuromas, and tumors near the ventricles,
    e.g., ependymomas. CSF protein in brainstem gliomas
    is generally normal. Encapsulated **brain abscesses**
    produce elevations similar to those seen in brain
    tumors.

3. **Spinal cord tumors** also raise protein levels, often
    to extremely high levels (e.g., 750 to 1000 mg/100
    ml), especially when block is present.

4. **Multiple sclerosis** may cause protein elevation in
    some patients, but the elevation is usually mild.
    Protein greater than 80 mg/100 ml in a patient with
    MS makes the diagnosis suspect.

5. **Acute purulent meningitis** invariably elevates the
    protein level regardless of the cause, as do subacute
    and chronic granulomatous meningitis. Viral
    infections of the CNS are associated with normal or
    mild increases in protein initially with a rise
    later, which serves as a clue to the diagnosis.
    Carcinomatous meningitis causes significant elevation
    of CSF protein.

6. **Infectious polyneuritis** (Guillain-Barré syndrome)
    characteristically causes increased protein levels.
    The protein is frequently normal during the first few
    days of the illness but rises after one week.

7. **Syphilis** produces increased protein levels in the
    meningovascular form and general paresis; the CSF may
    be normal in longstanding tabes.

8. Mild to moderate elevations may be seen in myxedema,
    uremia, connective tissue disorders, and Cushing's
    disease.

9. **Cerebrovascular disease** generally does not cause
    protein elevation, or only mild increases. There
    may, however, be large increases with cerebral
    hemorrhage because of serum protein in the CSF.

Gamma Globulin

The measurement of gamma globulin is used most
frequently to support the diagnosis of multiple sclerosis.

Normally, gamma globulin represents 13-15% or less of the total protein. (If total protein values are less than 20 mg/100 ml, the percentage of gamma globulin may be quite unreliable.) Gamma globulin is elevated in multiple sclerosis, subacute sclerosing panencephalitis, general paresis, herpes encephalitis, myxedema, some cases of carcinomatous cerebellar degeneration, and some connective tissue diseases. Measurement of IgG/albumin ratio (normally less than 0.18) provides similar information.

CSF Pressure

The CSF pressure is normally less than 200 mm H_2O with the patient lying (or at the level of the foramen magnum in the sitting position). It is not affected by changes in systemic blood pressure, but is exquisitely sensitive to changes in blood CO_2 (hyperventilation lowers intracranial pressure) and venous pressure.

1. Elevated pressures are seen in acute bacterial, fungal, and viral meningitis, or in meningoencephalitis.

2. There frequently is elevation with tumors or other intracerebral mass lesions (e.g., abscess), although pressure may be normal despite a large tumor.

3. Pressure is usually elevated in intracerebral bleeding and in subarachnoid hemorrhage.

4. Interestingly, the pressure and protein may be raised and there may be papilledema with polyneuritis or spinal tumor.

5. Unexplained elevated pressures may be due to congestive heart failure, chronic obstructive pulmonary disease (COPD), hypercapnia, jugular venous obstruction, or pericardial effusion.

6. Pseudotumor cerebri (benign raised intracranial pressure) refers to raised pressure, as high as 400 to 600 mm H_2O, with papilledema, not associated with a mass lesion or hydrocephalus, and with an otherwise normal CSF. Causes include: lateral venous sinus occlusion, withdrawal from steroids, pregnancy and menarche, hypo- or hypervitaminosis A, hyperparathyroidism, and tetracycline or phenothiazine administration. Female patients with

pseudotumor are frequently obese. Often the cause is unknown. One must first rule out tumor and hydrocephalus (usually with CAT scan) and then establish the diagnosis with LP. Lumbar punctures alone are often sufficient to lower CSF pressure and reverse the process. Acetazolamide may be given to decrease CSF production, and then steroids if necessary. Transient visual disturbances, such as blurring and dimming of vision are common in pseudotumor. More severe visual difficulties, such as field defects and actual loss of vision, can also occur and warrant vigorous treatment of the increased pressure, including lumbar peritoneal shunts and surgical decompression in protracted cases.

Pleocytosis

PMNs in the CSF suggest a bacterial infection, and lymphocytes a viral or chronic inflammatory process (although PMNs are sometimes seen at the onset of a viral infection). WBCs may be seen after subarachnoid hemorrhage, thrombosis, and, at times, with infectious mononucleosis; and eosinophils suggest a parasitic infection or dye reaction. Remember, many organic diseases of the CNS produce a mild pleocytosis. A thorough bacteriologic investigation must be carried out in all instances, even though cells do not always represent infection. Carcinomatous meningitis tends to be accompanied by less than 100 cells in the CSF (more than 100 cells suggests an infectious process). (Red cells are discussed in Chapter 5.)

REFERENCES

1. Fishman RA: Cerebrospinal Fluid in Diseases of the Nervous System. Philadelphia, Saunders, 1980.
2. Pearce JMS: Hazards of lumbar puncture. Brit Med J 285:1521, 1982.
3. Petito F, Plum F: The lumbar puncture. N Engl J Med 290:225, 1974.
4. Weisberg LA: Benign intracranial hypertension. Medicine 54:197, 1975.

Chapter 27

Neurodiagnostic Procedures

ELECTROENCEPHALOGRAM (EEG)

The EEG is a physiologic monitor of cerebral cortical function. It measures electrical activity which is generated in the cerebral cortex and then synchronized and modulated by thalamic and reticular activating structures. It is primarily a measure of gray matter or neuronal function and is abnormal when there is disease impinging on neurons or gray matter. The EEG is usually not abnormal in white matter disease.

1. Seizure Disorders

The EEG is a central test for the diagnosis and management of patients with seizure disorders. It should be emphasized that not all patients with clinically definite seizure disorders have abnormalities on EEG, and conversely, paroxysmal EEG abnormalities are sometimes seen in people without seizure disorders. During an actual seizure, an EEG usually demonstrates massive electrical discharge, followed in the postictal period by slowing. Interictal EEG's in patients with seizure disorders are abnormal in approximately 70% of patients. Certain seizure disorders are classified according to EEG patterns:

    a. Petit mal, a seizure characterized by brief
        losses of consciousness (e.g., staring spells of

no more than several seconds), occurs almost
exclusively between the ages of 5 and 18, and
shows classic 3 per second spike and wave
discharges. The diagnosis of petit mal depends on
that EEG finding.

b. Temporal lobe epilepsy is characterized by
focal EEG abnormalities in either or both
temporal lobes, including sharp waves or spike
discharges. These abnormalities may not be
apparent on routine interictal EEG's, but can
usually be demonstrated by sleep EEG's, or with
special nasopharyngeal or sphenoidal leads. If
temporal lobe epilepsy is suspected, such
procedures should be carried out.

The administration of anticonvulsants does not
necessarily affect the EEG, although certain medications
cause specific EEG patterns (e.g., barbiturates cause
Beta or fast wave patterns). Patients with a seizure
disorder who remain seizure-free for three to four years
and have an EEG which reverts to normal are usually taken
off medication. It is very important to remember in
treating people with seizure disorders that one must
"treat the patient" and not the EEG.

2. Cerebrovascular Disease. The EEG can be useful in
cerebrovascular disease in differentiating cortical
from subcortical strokes. In general, patients with
involvement of cortex secondary to large vessel
disease usually have abnormalities on EEG, while
small vessel subcortical or brainstem infarctions are
associated with normal EEG patterns. New onset of
seizures in old age is often a clinical clue for
unsuspected cerebrovascular disease.

3. Metabolic Encephalopathy. Patients with metabolic
encephalopathy of any cause have abnormal EEG's,
consisting of non-focal slowing of the EEG pattern or
rhythmic bursts of symmetrical frontal slowing. The
EEG can be useful in identifying metabolic
encephalopathies or in ruling out metabolic
encephalopathies in patients with altered mental
status. Sometimes these patterns can be quite
helpful, e.g., the "triphasic" waves of hepatic
encephalopathy.

4.   Tumors. Depending on the location and size of a
      tumor, the EEG is often abnormal, with either focal
      slowing or spike discharges. New onset of seizures
      in middle age is often the presenting symptom for
      tumor. However, the CAT scan is the major test used
      to diagnose tumors or other space-occupying lesions.

5.   Other Diseases. Surprisingly, the EEG may be
      normal in certain disorders which profoundly alter
      mental status (Alzheimer's disease, Wernicke-
      Korsakoff syndrome, delirium tremens). Some
      infectious disorders of the central nervous system do
      not affect the brain wave (e.g., cryptococcal
      meningitis), although others (e.g., Jacob-Creutzfeld
      disease, herpes simplex encephalitis) produce
      characteristic EEG changes. Psychiatric diseases
      (affective disorders, schizophrenia) have no effect
      on the EEG. Migraine headaches may be associated
      with focal slowing. Post-traumatic contusions may
      cause focal slowing or even paroxysmal activity.

   ELECTROMYOGRAPHY (EMG), NERVE CONDUCTION VELOCITY

A.   EMG

      The electromyogram (EMG) is an electrical test
measuring physiologic function in muscle. It is used to
help diagnose muscle disease, disease of the neuromuscular
junction, and denervation of muscles secondary to nerve or
root lesions.

1.   Myopathy. Patients with myopathy often show
      certain features: 1) low amplitude, short duration
      motor unit potentials; 2) polyphasic motor unit
      potentials; 3) increased insertional activity (e.g.,
      bizarre high frequency discharges). It is usually
      not possible to distinguish one myopathy from another
      by EMG. Some myopathies (e.g., polymyositis and
      muscular dystrophies) may show fibrillation
      potentials.

2.   Myotonia presents a characteristic pattern of
      hyperexcitability with persistent waxing and waning
      and repetitive discharges, which sound myographically
      like a "dive bomber". The dive bomber pattern is not
      diagnostic of any single myotonic disorder, but is
      characteristic of myotonia.

3. **Neuromuscular junction (NMJ) disorders.**
Pre-synaptic NMJ disorders (e.g., botulism,
Eaton-Lambert syndrome) may be characterized by
progressive enhancement of motor unit action
potentials evoked by repetitive stimulation of the
motor nerve; most also show normal amplitude
miniature end-plate potentials. By contrast,
post-synaptic NMJ disorders (e.g., myasthenia gravis)
show a decremental response of the muscle action
potential with repetitive nerve stimulation and
subnormal amplitudes of the miniature end-plate
potentials. Both pre- and post-synaptic EMG's show
increased **jitter** or variation in latency between a
nerve stimulus and the resulting muscle action
potentials.

4. **Denervation** produces increased polyphasic action
potentials, bizarre high frequency discharges,
fibrillations, positive sharp waves, and
fasciculations. Fibrillation potentials develop
three to four weeks after the onset of nerve injury.
Thus, someone with an acute root or nerve lesion may
not show muscle fibrillation. Examination of muscle
groups in the legs or arms may help diagnose specific
root lesions. Similarly, denervation can be used to
help diagnose ALS or other anterior horn cell
diseases. Disorders of the proximal nerve, including
the cell body, will prolong the "F response", which
is a peripherally recorded potential produced by
retrograde conduction of a stimulated action
potential to the soma with subsequent orthograde
conduction back to the periphery. The Hoffman or H
reflex is an orthograde motor potential generated by
stimulating sensory fibers in the stretch reflex arc.
Thus, an H reflex can be used to detect either
sensory or motor root lesions. The "F response" is
particularly useful in disorders which primarily
affect the proximal nerve (e.g., early stages of
Guillain-Barré syndrome).

B. **Nerve conduction velocities**

Nerve conduction velocities yield information as to
the integrity of both myelin and axon in peripheral nerve.
If nerve conduction velocity is slowed in all limbs, a
generalized neuropathy is implied (e.g., diabetic or
alcoholic neuropathies). Disorders which primarily affect

myelin (e.g., Guillain Barre) cause nerve conduction
slowing out of proportion to EMG changes, while "axonal"
neuropathies (e.g., due to alcohol) cause EMG changes of
denervation out of proportion to nerve conduction
abnormalities. Individual nerve abnormalities can be seen
in nerve entrapments (e.g., carpal tunnel) or nerve
infarction or damage (e.g., mononeuritis multiplex).

C.   Evoked Potentials

     An evoked potential is an electrical response
recorded from the central nervous system, elicited by an
external stimulus -- visual, auditory, or somatosensory.
Evoked potentials are useful in localizing subtle sensory
lesions and in detecting unsuspected subclinical sensory
deficits.

1.   Visual evoked responses (VER's), measured over the
     occiput, are stimulated by flashing lights or
     shifting checkerboard patterns in the visual fields.
     They are most helpful in demonstrating lesions in the
     optic nerves and are particularly useful in the
     diagnosis of multiple sclerosis. The majority of
     patients with a history of optic neuritis or multiple
     sclerosis have VER abnormalities. VER changes are
     also seen in toxic and nutritional amblyopias, tumors
     compressing the anterior visual pathways, Friedrich's
     ataxia, and pernicious anemia. VER's may also be of
     benefit in patients suspected of hysterical visual
     loss. They are also helpful in monitoring optic
     nerve and chiasm function in patients with pituitary
     tumors or pseudotumor cerebri.

2.   Brainstem auditory evoked responses (BAER's) are
     elicited by delivering click stimuli to either ear.
     Their major advantage is the ability to localize
     auditory pathway lesions to 8th nerve, cochlear
     nucleus, superior olive, lateral lemniscus, or
     inferior colliculus. They are exquisitely sensitive
     to extrinsic lesions such as acoustic neuromas, and
     may detect these lesions before they are visible by
     CAT scan. They are also sensitive to intrinsic
     brainstem lesions impinging on the auditory pathways,
     seen in multiple sclerosis, brainstem glioma,
     brainstem infarcts, and olivopontocerebellar
     degeneration. Because they are not abolished by high

doses of anesthesia or barbiturates, they are useful
monitors of brainstem integrity in patients rendered
comatose or treated with these agents. They may
prove useful as prognostic indicators in the comatose
patient, especially after head trauma.

3.   Somatosensory evoked responses (SER's) are elicited
      by stimulating large fiber sensory systems
      peripherally. Tibial and peroneal evoked responses
      may help localize lesions to their respective
      peripheral nerves, lumbo-sacral plexus, dorsal spinal
      cord, spino-medullary junction, brainstem and
      thalamus. Median nerve SER's will assess function
      across Erb's point, and centrally through
      spino-medullary junction, brainstem and thalamus.
      Pudendal SER's help detect deficits of sensory
      innervation of the genitalia. Virtually any lesion
      compromising conduction in these systems (e.g.,
      multiple sclerosis, spinal cord tumors, severe
      spondylosis) may produce SER abnormalities. SER's
      are useful adjuncts to monitor spinal cord function
      during cord surgery.

                        CAT SCAN

     Computerized axial tomography clearly has provided a
revolution in the diagnosis and management of neurologic
disease. A complete review of findings on CAT scan is
beyond the scope of the manual. Nonetheless, certain
basic points should be kept in mind:

     Use of contrast in CAT scanning. CAT scans need
not necessarily be done with contrast enhancement, and
that decision should depend on the clinical situation.
Contrast enhancement is generally used to assist diagnosis
of demyelinating disease, infarctions, certain infections,
tumors, and vascular malformations, including aneurysms.
The danger of "routine" contrast use relates to allergy to
the dye and the effect of dye on renal function.

1.   Cerebrovascular disease. The basic value of the
      CAT scan in cerebrovascular disease is to
      differentiate hemorrhage from infarction. Virtually
      all hemorrhages show up as increased density on CAT
      scans, while either no abnormalities or decreased
      density are seen with infarction. This distinction

is of particular importance when it is impossible to distinguish infarction from hemorrhage on clinical grounds alone, since treatment is drastically different with these two conditions. No patient should be anticoagulated without prior CAT scan and/or lumbar puncture to rule out bleeding. Lumbar puncture is not as sensitive as CAT scan in identifying intracranial hemorrhage (see p. 24). Fifteen to 20% of infarcts are apparent immediately on CAT scan, and the majority of moderate-sized infarcts are apparent at 10-14 days. The diagnosis of multiple infarcts due to emboli can also be made by CAT scan, including infarcts seen in areas that have not declared themselves clinically. CAT scan can identify ateriovenous malformations and aneurysms, although the precise diagnosis of these disorders requires arteriography.

2.   Tumors. Virtually all tumors greater than 2-4 mm can be seen on CAT scan. Depending on the pattern, certain diagnostic interpretations can be made. CAT scan sensitivity to tumors is enhanced by perfusion with iodinated contrast agents.

3.   Hydrocephalus. The CAT scan has replaced pneumocephalography for the demonstration and evaluation of hydrocephalus.

4.   Degenerative diseases. Patients with CNS degenerative diseases, such as Alzheimer's disease, usually have abnormal CAT scans. However, as patients get older they usually have widened sulci and enlarged ventricles due to loss of brain tissue. Increase in depth of sulci does not necessarily correlate with dementia and can also be seen in "normal" people. There are patients with degenerative disease or dementia who have normal appearing CAT scans.

5.   Demyelinating disease. In a small percentage of patients with demyelinating disease, abnormalities may be seen on CAT scan. Periventricular white matter lesions may be well visualized, especially if carried out with contrast.

6.   Subdural hematoma. Approximately 80% of subdural hematomas, both unilaterally and bilaterally, can be

seen on CAT scan. Some subdurals may be isodense and not visualized by CAT scan and require arteriography or brain scan for diagnosis.

7.   **Brainstem and spinal cord**. It is possible to visualize sections of brainstem using advanced CAT scans and contrast enhancement. Thus, increasingly, one can diagnose acoustic neuroma, pontine gliomas, and large arteriovenous malformations. CAT scanning of spinal cord is improving rapidly. It can be used for diagnosis of disc disease and tumor metastases, but is limited by the fact that one cannot image the entire spinal cord in horizontal sections by CT. Thus, spinal CAT scans should be reserved for clinical situations in which the exam suggests a specific spinal level.

8.   **Trauma**. CAT scan is effective in differentiating a wide variety of consequences of trauma in the nervous system, including fractures, epidural and subdural hematomas, and shifts of intracranial contents. CAT scan is an excellent screening method to show intracranial shifts prior to performing lumbar puncture.

NUCLEAR MAGNETIC RESONANCE

This rapidly evolving form of neuro-imaging offers a new dimension in the visualization of lesions. It is presently beginning to be evaluated in clinical trials. NMR appears to be very good at delineating lesions not formerly seen, such as plaques in multiple sclerosis, and visualization of spinal cord lesions. NMR works by magnetic excitation of atoms and thus offers the benefit of no X-ray exposure.

ARTERIOGRAPHY

Cerebral arteriography is used to define vascular disease of both intracranial and extracranial vessels, e.g., carotid artery disease, arteriovenous malformation, and aneurysms. Digital venous angiography allows computer-enhanced views of the carotid arteries without the risk of arteriography.

REFERENCES

1.   Chiappa KH, Ropper AH: Evoked potentials in
      clinical medicine. N Engl J Med 306:1140, 1205,
      1982.
2.   Goodgold J, Eberstein A: Electrodiagnosis of
      Neuromuscular Diseases. Baltimore, Williams &
      Wilkins, 1972.
3.   Kilch LG, McComas AJ, Osselton JW: Clinical
      Electroencephalography, 4th ed, London, Butterworth,
      1978.
4.   Lee SH, Rao KC: Cranial Computed Tomography. New
      York, McGraw-Hill, 1982.

Chapter 28

Neuroanatomy

CIRCLE OF WILLIS

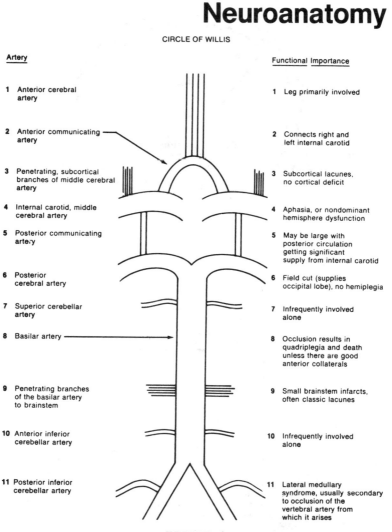

Artery

1 Anterior cerebral artery

2 Anterior communicating artery

3 Penetrating, subcortical branches of middle cerebral artery

4 Internal carotid, middle cerebral artery

5 Posterior communicating artery

6 Posterior cerebral artery

7 Superior cerebellar artery

8 Basilar artery

9 Penetrating branches of the basilar artery to brainstem

10 Anterior inferior cerebellar artery

11 Posterior inferior cerebellar artery

Functional Importance

1 Leg primarily involved

2 Connects right and left internal carotid

3 Subcortical lacunes, no cortical deficit

4 Aphasia, or nondominant hemisphere dysfunction

5 May be large with posterior circulation getting significant supply from internal carotid

6 Field cut (supplies occipital lobe), no hemiplegia

7 Infrequently involved alone

8 Occlusion results in quadriplegia and death unless there are good anterior collaterals

9 Small brainstem infarcts, often classic lacunes

10 Infrequently involved alone

11 Lateral medullary syndrome, usually secondary to occlusion of the vertebral artery from which it arises

FIGURE 4

EYE DEVIATION IN NEUROLOGIC DISEASE

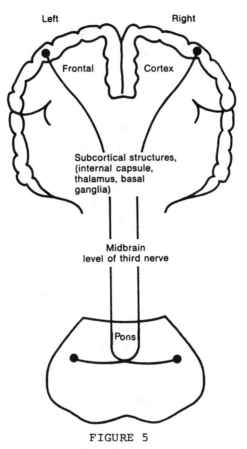

FIGURE 5

Note: The frontal eye fields exert a major
influence on horizontal eye movement, each field being
concerned with contralateral eye deviation. Thus, the
right field causes eyes to move to the left. (The fibers
cross in the pons and there connect to the extraocular
muscles via the medial longitudinal fasciculus.) Both
fields are constantly active, striking a balance; thus,
when one is more or less active than the other, horizontal
eye deviation results.

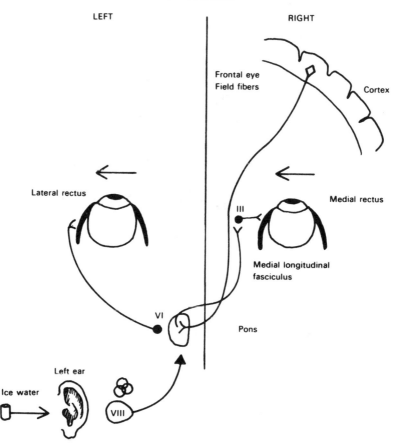

FIGURE 6

In the comatose patient with an intact brainstem, ice water in the left ear causes deviation of the eyes to the left. In the awake patient, this deviation is counteracted voluntarily, producing nystagmus to the right.

A <u>destructive lesion</u> in the hemisphere or subcortex causes eyes to deviate toward the same side as the lesion.   Thus, with a right-sided lesion the eyes are deviated to the right.   An <u>excitatory lesion</u> at the cortical level (viz, a seizure) causes eyes to deviate to the contralateral side.   Thus, with a left-sided seizure eyes are driven to the right.   A <u>destructive lesion</u> in the pons (after fibers have crossed) causes eyes to deviate to the side opposite the damage.   Thus, with a left-sided lesion eyes deviate to the right.   (There are no excitatory lesions of the pons.)   Eye deviation secondary to hemisphere lesions, but not brainstem lesions, may be overcome by brainstem reflexes, e.g., doll's eyes maneuver.

VISUAL PATHWAY

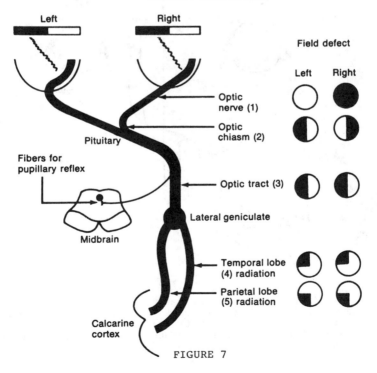

FIGURE 7

1. <u>Blindness in one eye</u> represents retinal or optic
    nerve dysfunction. The optic nerve is frequently
    involved in multiple sclerosis (optic neuritis),
    producing unilateral blindness; it may also be
    involved by tumor (optic glioma) or undergo atrophy
    secondary to prolonged raised intracranial pressure.
    The optic nerve may also be affected by vascular
    processes such as giant cell arteritis and amaurosis
    fugax.

2. <u>Bitemporal hemianopsia</u> is classically found in
    pituitary tumors secondary to pressure on the optic
    chiasm. Non-homonymous field defects usually imply a
    chiasmal lesion. Remember that concentric tunnel
    vision may be seen in hysterical blindness.

3. <u>Homonymous hemianopsia</u> implies a lesion posterior
    to the chiasm. It may involve optic tract or optic
    radiations emanating from the lateral geniculate body
    (or the lateral geniculate itself). The closer a
    lesion is to the lateral geniculate, the smaller it
    can be and still produce a homonymous hemianopsia.

4. The <u>optic radiations</u> fan out from the lateral
    geniculate and travel in the temporal and parietal
    lobes before reaching their destination in the
    occipital lobe. Lesions in the temporal lobe may
    give a homonymous superior field defect if the optic
    radiations are affected. Similarly, a lesion in the
    parietal lobe may show an inferior homonymous field
    defect.

5. The <u>pupillary response</u> is affected only if fibers
    proximal to the lateral geniculate body, in the
    midbrain, third nerve or optic nerve fibers are
    damaged.

6. When one realizes the large territory needed for
    intact visual fields, it becomes apparent why
    checking visual fields is a mandatory part of every
    neurologic examination.

SPINAL CORD

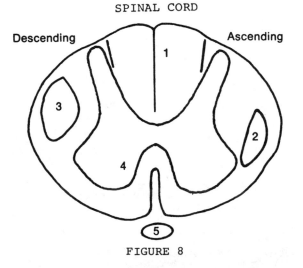

FIGURE 8

Ascending Tracts

Dorsal columns (1) carry position and vibratory sense; fibers rise ipsilaterally and cross in the medulla. These columns are laminated, but the lamination is usually of little clinical importance.

Lateral spinothalamic tract (2) carries pain and temperature sensation. These fibers cross upon entering the cord; a cord lesion affecting them produces a contralateral loss. They are laminated with sacral fibers most laterally placed. Thus, an expanding process in the center of the cord gives sacral sparing (pinprick and temperature sensory loss are least prominent in the sacral area).

Descending Tracts

Lateral corticospinal tract (3) carries motor fibers which synapse at the anterior horn cells. The fibers have already crossed in the medulla. A lesion of or pressure upon the corticospinal tract causes weakness, spasticity, hyperreflexia, and upgoing toes.

Anterior horn cells (4) are lower motor neurons. A lesion here produces weakness, muscle wasting, fasciculations, and loss of reflexes and tone.

Vascular Supply

The **anterior spinal artery** (5) supplies the entire
cord except for the dorsal columns. Thus, the anterior
spinal artery syndrome produces paralysis and loss of pain
and temperature sense; position and vibratory sense are
preserved.

Clinical Correlation

- Combined system disease affects 1 and 3

- Amyotrophic lateral sclerosis affects 3 and 4

- Tabes dorsalis affects 1

- Multiple sclerosis affects 1, 2, and 3
  (alone or in combination)

- Poliomyelitis affects 4

- Brown-Séquard syndrome (hemisection of cord)
  produces ipsilateral paralysis and contralateral
  loss of sensation to pinprick

MEDULLA (Cranial Nerves 9 to 12)

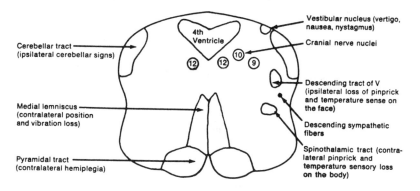

FIGURE 9

The most commonly encountered vascular syndrome
affecting the medulla is the <u>lateral medullary
(Wallenberg) syndrome</u> (see chapter 6), which defines a
major portion of the dysfunction that can be seen with
medullary involvement. (Medial structures are not
affected: pyramids, medial lemniscus, and twelfth nerve
nucleus.)

Remember that the <u>seventh</u> (facial) <u>nerve is not
in the medulla</u>; thus, if facial weakness is present,
there must be dysfunction at the level of the pons or
above.

When <u>descending sympathetic fibers</u> are involved,
an ipsilateral Horner's syndrome (ptosis, small pupil,
and facial anhidrosis) results.

<u>Cranial nerve nuclei</u>:

- . <u>Twelfth</u> (hypoglossal): Unilateral involvement
    of nucleus causes fasciculations on that side;
    when the tongue is protruded it deviates to the
    side of the lesion.

- . <u>Tenth</u> (vagus) and <u>ninth</u> (glossopharyngeal):
    these innervate the laryngeal and pharyngeal
    musculature; dysphagia is prominent when they are
    involved.

PONS (Cranial Nerves 5 to 8)

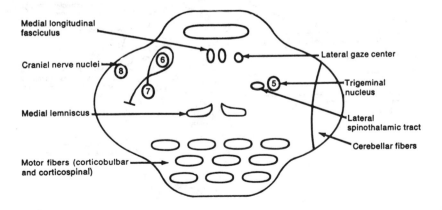

FIGURE 10

The fibers of the seventh (facial) nerve sweep around the sixth nerve (lateral rectus) before exiting from the pons. Thus a lesion at this level often produces a VI and VII nerve paralysis on the same side.

Basic structure of the pons: Medial involvement produces motor dysfunction and internuclear ophthalmoplegia or gaze palsy to the side of the lesion. Lateral involvement causes pain and temperature dysfunction.

Vertical nystagmus is a sign of brainstem dysfunction at the level of the pontomedullary junction or upper midbrain (unless the patient is on barbiturates).

Eighth nerve nuclei include cochlear and vestibular components.

The trigeminal nerve exits from the middle of the pons and if involved at this level produces face pain and ipsilateral loss of the corneal reflex. In high pontine lesions pain and sensory loss are contralateral to the lesion in both face and extremities. Below the high pons, pain and temperature senses are lost ipsilaterally in the face and contralaterally in the limbs.

Lesions of the medial longitudinal fasciculus (MLF) result in an internuclear ophthalmoplegia. If the right MLF is involved, there is difficulty with right eye adduction, as well as nystagmus in the abducting left eye when the patient looks to the left.

The most prominent disturbance in the midbrain generally involves the third nerve nucleus or exiting fibers, producing a dilated pupil and ophthalmoplegia.

MIDBRAIN (Cranial Nerves 3 to 4)

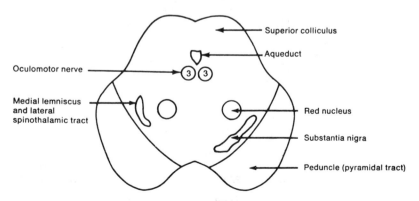

FIGURE 11

Lesions affecting the area of the midbrain just below the superior colliculus produce difficulty with upward gaze convergence and pupillary light reflexes (Parinaud's syndrome). A tumor pressing on the superior colliculus may present in this way (e.g., pinealoma).

Lesions of the red nucleus produce contralateral ataxia and tremor (rubral tremor). The substantia nigra is located at this level and plays an important role in Parkinson's disease.

The fourth nerve nucleus is also located in the midbrain at a lower level and is seldom involved alone. When it is involved alone (e.g., due to trauma), fourth nerve injury causes a head tilt.

Fibers from the optic tract concerned with the pupillary response synapse in the region of the third nerve nucleus. Lesions in the midbrain may impair pupillary reaction to direct light, but leave contraction to accommodation intact.

DERMATOME SENSORY CHART

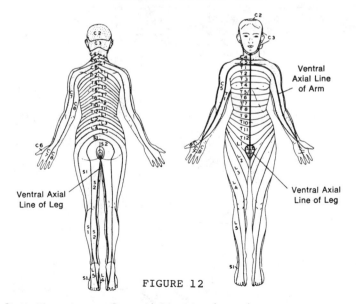

FIGURE 12

Left: Dermatomes from the posterior view.
Right: The dermatomes from the anterior view.   From Keegan JJ and Garrett FD: The segmental distribution of the cutaneous nerves in the limbs of man. <u>Anat. Rec.</u> 102: 409, 1948. Reprinted by permission of the Wistar Institute Press, Philadelphia, Pennsylvania.

CROSSINGS IN THE NERVOUS SYSTEM

Almost all major pathways in the nervous system cross. Much of the understanding of neuroanatomy relates to knowing where these tracts cross and thus at which level the nervous system is involved.

Pathway	Function	Crosses	Interpretation
Pyramidal tract	Motor	Lower medulla	Lesion below crossing gives ipsilateral signs
Spino-thalamic tract	Pain and temperature (body)	On entry to spinal cord	Lesion is always contra-lateral to pain and temperature loss (except in face)
Spinal tract of fifth (V) nerve	Pain and temperature (face)	Midpons (runs through-out medulla)	If lesion is in medulla or lower pons - ipsilateral loss; above mid-pons - contralat-eral loss
Spinal dorsal columns	Position and vibration	Lower medulla	Lesion below crossing gives ipsilateral signs
Cere-bellar tracts	Coordina-tion of movement	Crosses twice (on entry to cerebellum and in midbrain)	Because of the "double cross-ing" lesions of cerebellum or cerebellar tracts usually produce signs and symptoms ipsilateral to lesion

(continued on following page)

CROSSINGS IN THE NERVOUS SYSTEM (cont'd.)

Pathway	Function	Crosses	Interpretation
Gaze fibers	Coordinates lateral gaze	Midpons	See Fig. 5 for interpretation
Cranial nerve fibers	Cranial nerves	Just above cranial nerve nuclei	Lesion is ipsilateral when cranial nerve nuclei are involved

Index